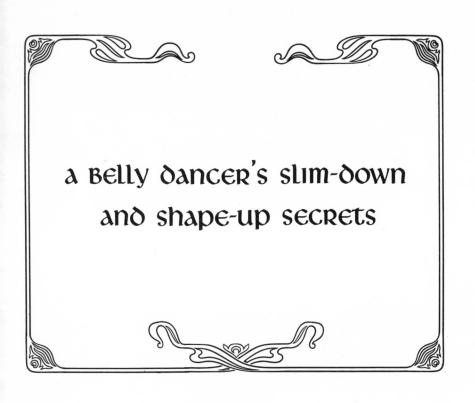

a belly dancer's slim-down and shape-up secrets

a Belly Dancer's slim-down and shape-up secrets

by Lebwa

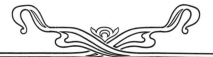

Parker Publishing Company, Inc.
West Nyack, New York

© 1979 *by*

PARKER PUBLISHING COMPANY, INC.

West Nyack, N.Y.

This book is a reference work based on research by the author. The opinions expressed herein are not necessarily those of or endorsed by the publisher. The directions stated in this book are in no way to be considered as a substitute for consultation with a duly licensed doctor.

Library of Congress Cataloging in Publication Data

Lebwa,
    A belly dancer's slim-down and shape-up secrets.

    Includes index.
    1. Reducing. 2. Reducing diets--Recipes. 3. Cookery, Near East. 4. Reducing exercises. 5. Belly dance. I. Title.
RM222.2.L38   613.2'5   79-12771
ISBN 0-13-074906-0

Printed in the United States of America

Dedication

To my daughter, Cathy, who can finally stop going around the house asking, "Is this book ever going to be finished?"

How This Book Will Make You Slimmer and Shapelier

In order for your body to be slim, shapely, completely healthy, and truly beautiful you must begin to nurture it from inside. This book was written to help you achieve that internal beauty and subsequently an outward beauty for the rest of your life. As an experienced belly dancer I am engaged in an exotic, stimulating dance form, and I have discovered that we dancers have some fascinating secrets of a happy, healthy, exciting life without knowing it. I am also a New York public school teacher, and as a teacher, I feel I have to share my knowledge. Thus *A Belly Dancer's Slim-Down and Shape-Up Secrets* is my way of showing you how you can have the beautiful figure of a professional dancer. This book is going to show you a delightful way to embark on a new way of life, and I would like you to keep it as a reference to guide you for a long time to come.

I'm sure that if you are overweight you want to do something about the extra weight that you are carrying about. This book will also show you how to maintain your weight if you are already blessed with a great figure. I know you also want to lead a healthy, happy life. My "secrets" will help you to achieve this goal in a fascinating, exotic way.

I have developed a very simple plan that will make you healthier and happier and that you will be able to follow without any problems. As a belly dancer I have to watch what I eat very carefully, so I have gone about dieting in a simple way that would give me the most flexibility and at the same time not bore me to death. My eating plan features the exotic and delicious foods of the Middle East.

Belly dancing is such a lot of fun that you may end up wanting to become a professional dancer, but for most people it is simply a wonderful help in shedding excess pounds or in tightening up and maintaining an already svelte shape. You won't have to be bored with dull exercises, since you will find yourself enlivened by a stimulating activity in a pleasant atmosphere which will take off your pounds before you even know it. Moreover, with my approach you will be discovering a whole new culture while you are shedding a lot of excess weight.

All of my belly dance exercises are done to music, which helps to soothe ruffled nerves and calm the stressful days that we all have sometimes. You will have a variety of dance-related movements for each part of your body from which to choose, and as you dance, you'll float off to a faraway continent and perhaps even to another period in time if you really concentrate and let your imagination run away with you.

My exercises would not be worth the paper on which they are printed if I didn't also provide a well-balanced eating plan. All the exotic dances in the world would do you absolutely no good if you continued to stuff your body. Instead, I'm going to give you a balanced diet. You will enjoy delicious foods providing each of the six essential nutrients that you need to have a healthy and attractive body.

The eating pattern that I am suggesting lets you eat virtually anything you like. This "diet" is easy to maintain, even when you are dining with the Queen of England. You are going to learn to eat the Middle Eastern way and lose pounds at the same time. You will also learn how to make and enjoy delightful low-calorie Middle Eastern dishes. What a tasty way to slim down!

Without a doubt, the belly dance can do wonders for you. It has been called a sexy, sensuous dance, and that is not merely by accident. (And what book today would be complete without some advice on how to improve your sex life?) Most belly dancers have tried to maintain that sensuous quality, but today they are going beyond that and broadening the scope of the dance to include elements of many folk dances. I'll guide you through a short history of the belly dance, both Turkish and Arabic versions, while you slim down and shape up.

I'm taking you on a pilgrimage—a long delightful journey to health and beauty, traveling in your imagination down the waters of the Nile River. Then you'll transfer yourself from that body of water to your bathtub, where you'll embark on some magnificent water exercises to help your body keep fit. I'll show you how to make your bath a sensuous, healthy part of your life.

After you have reached your goal, I'm going to explain how you can show off your new figure to all your friends at a smashing Arabian Nights extravaganza. I am going to show you how to turn your house into an Arabian Nights fantasyland. Finally, I am going to tell you how to embark on a lifetime of physical fitness that belly dancers enjoy.

Your horizons will be broadened, your bodies will be tightened, and your mind will be stretched beyond your imagination. So read and enjoy as I guide you through this experience, step-by-step, the belly dancer's way. Come now with me on an exotic pilgrimage to a beautiful, healthy, slim, and shapely body.

Lebwa

ACKNOWLEDGMENTS

I wish to thank the following people for permission to reprint excerpts from their published works:

●Mr. Juan Metzger, Chairman of the Board of Dannon Milk Products, L.I.C., N.Y. for his kind help and advice: *Dieting, Yogurt and Common Sense*, Dannon 1975; *Yogurt and Gelatine*; *Yogurt and You* © 1976 Dannon Milk Products, Division of Beatrice Foods Co.

●*The Whirling Dervishes* by Ira Friedlander, with contributions by Nezih Uzel (Copyright © 1975 by Ira Friedlander).

●*The Best Foods of Russia*, copyright © 1976, by Sonia Uvezian, Harcourt Brace Jovanovich, Inc.

●Ruth Lundgren, Ltd. P.O. Box 184, Baldwin, N.Y. 11510 for the *Angostura Aromatic Bitters*.

●C P C International, International Plaza, Englewood Cliffs, N.J. 07632 for its Hellmann's Real Mayonnaise recipes.

●*The Wisdom of Gibran*, edited by Joseph Sheban, Philosophical Library, Inc. 15 East 40th Street, New York 10016 © Copyright, 1966.

●Ibrahim Farrah, publisher of *Arabesqué, A Journal of Middle Eastern Dance and Culture*, Ibrahim Farrah, Inc., New York for inspiration derived from his journal.

A book like this is the culmination of many people's influences on my life. It would be impossible for me to thank everyone who has touched my life in some way, so I will just say thanks to all my wonderful friends who have helped me along the way—they know who they are. How does one thank one's mother? Thanks Mom for everything.

Special gratitude goes to Dorothy Knowles, a dear friend whose knowledge of the Middle East and life in general I have admired for more years than I care to enumerate. Her help and advice with my manuscript are deeply appreciated.

Thanks also to Margaret Nelson, the talented artist at the Fernwood Hotel, Bushkill, Pennsylvania, who did the illustrations and put up so nicely with my impatience at holding indefinite poses for the exercises.

contents

**Making Yourself Familiar with Your Body's Needs
and Capabilities (cont.)**

**5. The Easy Way to Limber Up and Begin
Oriental Dancing** 103

6. How a Pita a Day Keeps the Pounds and Inches Away 134

**7. How to Bring Each Part of Your Body to Life in
Oriental Dancing** 148

How to Bring Each Part of Your Body to Life in Oriental Dancing (cont.)

**Keeping the Health and Beauty of an Oriental
Dancer All Your Life (cont.)**

Appendix **314**

Index **332**

METRIC CONVERSION OF MEASUREMENTS USED

Volume

teaspoons	multiply by 5 to get *milliliters*
tablespoons	multiply by 15 to get *milliliters*
cups	multiply by 24 to get *liters*
pints	multiply by 47 to get *liters*
quarts	multiply by 95 to get *liters*

Mass (weight)

ounces	multiply by 28 to get *grams*
pounds	multiply by 45 to get *kilograms*

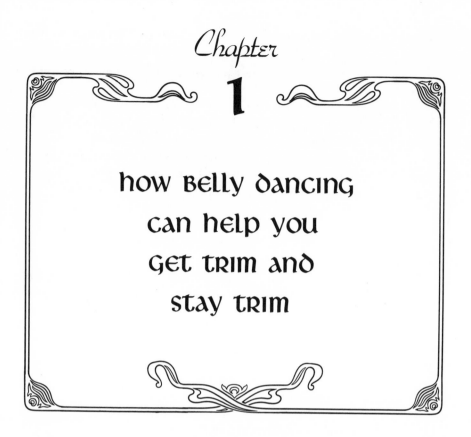

Chapter 1

how belly dancing can help you get trim and stay trim

Belly dancing is one of the easiest and most pleasant ways by which you can give yourself a new figure, and lose weight. Many belly dancers have been known to lose as much as four pounds during a single performance. The belly dancing you will learn in this book will enable you to shed pounds without setting foot on a stage.

The belly dance, or Oriental dance, is probably the oldest form of dance in existence. It is a beautiful, healthy, and sensuous dance when done correctly. The dance is misnamed "belly dance" because it uses all parts of the body—actually the term came from *belledi dance*, "belledi" being an Arabic word meaning village or country. In the Middle East, both men and women do these dances.

You are going to learn belly dance steps and movements in the form of easy, pleasant exercises. They are very simple and straightforward. Anyone will be able to do them, and you will find that you will have so much fun you'll forget you are exercising. They will soon be a natural part of your daily routine for health and beauty.

You'll love your belly dance exercises for the following reasons:

1. You don't need any special ability to do these exercises.
2. They can be performed without any special equipment.
3. They will generally improve your physical fitness.
4. Because they are such fun, you will continue to be motivated.
5. They will wipe away any stress and tension, and you will get a feeling of well-being from them.
6. They will "turn you on" to a new and fascinating world—the world of the Middle East.
7. They will open your mind to new experiences.

As you may know, you expend energy even in as simple an exercise as walking. Dancing uses even more energy, burning up excess fat and strengthening your muscles. At the same time it is soothing and relaxing. You will discover that belly dance exercises will benefit all parts of your body. Whether you are a man or woman, these exercises will:

—improve your posture.
—improve your breathing.
—improve your blood circulation.
—loosen your tense muscles.
—tighten your flabby muscles.
—improve your general appearance.
—help you overcome stress and nervous tension.
—soothe your emotions.
—help prevent heart attacks and other diseases.

Over all, belly dancing will make you feel like a new person. Before you begin any exercise and diet program you should, of course, check with your doctor to be sure you are in good physical condition. Otherwise there is no need for undue concern because you will not hurt yourself if you do the exercises slowly and carefully as you are directed.

WARM-UP EXERCISES

As with any exercise program, it is important to prepare your body for the changes it will go through during your exercises. Therefore it will be necessary to limber up or "warm up" your body before you start your belly dancing. Following are four simple "warm-up" stretches to help you get underway. Do these body stretches as directed before you try any of the belly dance exercises.

Warm-Up Exercise #1
Wrist Stretch

- Assume correct posture.
- Hands at sides.
- Slowly raise arms to shoulder level, straight out in front, palms face down.
- Bend hands at wrists, hold fingers straight down.
- Hold for a count of 5, relax.
- Repeat twice.
- Increase to a count of 10 after a few days.
- Bend hands at wrists, hold fingers straight up.
- Hold for a count of 5.
- Repeat twice.
- Increase to a count of 10 after a few days.

Warm-Up Exercise #2
Circular Neck Stretches

- Assume correct posture.
- Hands at sides.
- Relax completely, eyes closed.
- Swing head over to the left shoulder until ear almost touches your shoulder.
- Start slowly rotating head in a circular clockwise direction.
- Take four counts until head is lowered in front and chin is tucked into the chest.
- Take four counts to swing head over to the right shoulder.
- Take four counts to swing head back (back of head should touch middle of shoulderblade).
- Then take four counts to swing head over to the left shoulder.
- Altogether this should take you a slow count of 16 to make a complete circle.
- Repeat twice, relax.

- Do the same thing counterclockwise twice.
- This stretch exercise can be done either in a standing or a seated position.

Warm-Up Exercise #3
Waist and Torso Stretch

- Assume correct posture.
- Hands at sides.
- Slowly raise both hands until they are straight up overhead.
- Slowly reach up with the right hand and stretch as far as you can as if reaching for something on a high shelf.
- Hold for a count of 5.
- Increase to a count of 10 after a few days.
- Slowly return hand to side.
- Slowly reach up with the left hand and stretch as far as you can.
- Hold for a count of 5.
- Increase to a count of 10 after a few days.
- Slowly return hand to side.
- Alternate hands.
- Repeat 5 times.

Warm-Up Exercise #4
Back Stretch (seated)

- Assume seated position.
- Feet straight out in front.
- Hands at sides.
- Slowly raise arms to shoulder level.
- Lower arms to calves and hold calves with hands.
- Lower head as close to thighs as possible.
- Hold for a count of 5.
- Increase to a count of 10 after a few days.
- Repeat 5 times.

ASSUMING CORRECT POSTURE

Let me say just a word about correct posture. Too many people just seem to slump all over. So many of my friends do—indeed, I am guilty of this too and have to catch myself at times. This kind of sluggish sitting and standing is most detrimental to the body.

The following is the correct posture that you should assume for all exercises. When I say, "Assume correct posture," you should hold your body in the following position:

1. Head straight up, chin tucked in
2. Shoulders straight
3. Breastbone up
4. Pelvis straight under trunk
5. Knees bent slightly
6. Feet slightly apart
7. Hands at your sides
8. Your position should be one of ease, do not strain yourself.

To achieve correct posture it isn't necessary to "lock" your body into a stiff, unnatural pose. It is necessary to see that every part of your body is functioning the way it is supposed to function. If your head was meant to hang loosely, drooping down to your chest, then it would have been set in that position. Until you need to use it in that position, you should keep it straight up and keep your chin tucked in.

BEGINNER'S EXERCISES

Now try the simple "beginner's" belly dance exercises that I have included here so that you can see how quickly you can start getting trim and having some fun. They will take you only about 10 minutes a day to get you in the mood to go on to bigger and better things later on. Even grandmothers in the Middle East do this dance all the time without a problem, and so can you.

Eye Isolation

- Assume correct posture.
- Raise hands and arms to shoulder level.
- Bend elbows and bring hands in front of nose, palms touch facing downwards.
- Hands one on top of the other.
- Slowly roll eyes over to the left as far as you can.
- Slowly roll eyes to the right as far as you can.
- Repeat 5 times.

The eyes are one of the most neglected parts of the body in most exercise programs. This is a shame because all parts of your body need exercise. Besides the exercise value here, this simple eye movement is one of the most sensual ones used in the belly dance. Your eyes can speak for you as well as the spoken word. Dancers often use the veil to isolate and bring attention to their eyes. This is done by draping the veil around the head so that only the eyes are exposed.

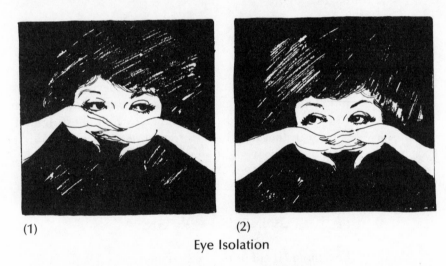

(1)   (2)

Eye Isolation

Slow Stomach Flutter

- Assume correct posture.
- Hands down at sides.
- Slowly pull in and tense stomach muscles as if someone pushed you in the stomach—breathe in.
- Hold for a count of 2.

- Release and relax stomach muscles to their original position—breathe out.
- Hold for a count of 2.
- Repeat this in and out movement 10 times.
- After several weeks this slow flutter can be speeded up so that you achieve a beautiful effect in your stomach area.

You will soon find that this exercise can be a very beneficial one for the stomach muscles. The stomach is another area of the body that is frequently neglected, and the first sign of a weight problem usually manifests itself in this area. Several variations of this exercise are used in preparation for natural childbirth.

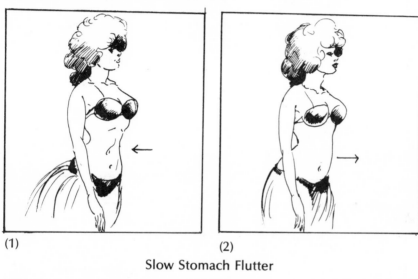

(1)   (2)

Slow Stomach Flutter

Single Arm Circles

- Assume correct posture.
- Start with arms by your sides.
- Bring left arm in front of your stomach.
- Slowly swing left arm up and out to the side.
- Stretch your arm out at shoulder level and continue raising the arm until it comes over your head, fingers pointing to the ceiling.
- Bring elbow over in front of your face.
- Complete the circle by bringing arm down in front of you.
- Return arm to your side.
- Repeat 3 times.

- Do the same circular movement with the right hand.
- Repeat 3 times.

The arm movements in the belly dance can make or break a dancer's performance. They must be graceful; otherwise they look like the mechanically stiff arms of a robot. Arms often develop unsightly "flab." By exercising your arms regularly you are going to bring new tone and control into them, making that flab disappear.

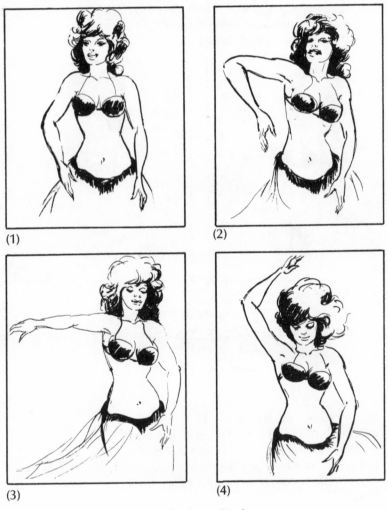

(1)   (2)

(3)   (4)

Single Arm Circles

Wrist Rubs or Slides

- Assume correct posture.
- Bring arms up to shoulder level.
- Bring hands up to a praying position in front of your chest.
- Press your wrists together.
- Slowly rub the wrists against each other in a fan-like motion.

This exercise can be done either standing or in a seated position. To add variety, the hands can be held just about any place you desire to hold them.

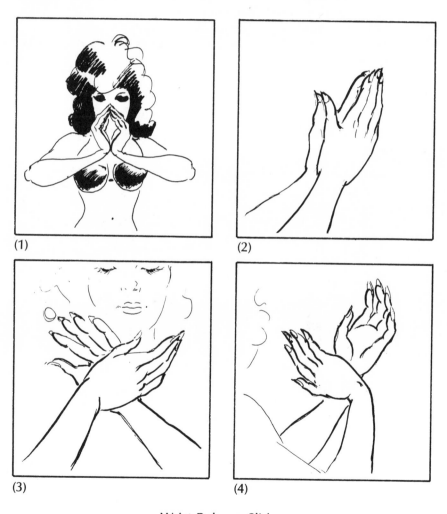

(1)

(2)

(3)

(4)

Wrist Rubs or Slides

Belly Dance Basic Step

- Assume correct posture.
- Stand straight, feet slightly apart, left foot in front of right foot.
- Step flat on the right foot and tap with the ball of the left foot, thrusting your hip out to the side at the same time.
- Step flat on the left foot and tap with the ball of the right foot, thrusting your hip out to the side at the same time.
- Keep your knees bent, your body relaxed, and hold your hands above your head in a graceful pose.
- Twist your body from side to side on the tap step.
- You can do this exercise in one place or you can travel around the room with it.
- Repeat for about 2 minutes.

This is the basic "travelling" step that dancers use to move around the stage. As in all our dance steps, you can use many variations. For example, try thrusting the pelvis gently forward instead of thrusting the hip sidewards as you move.

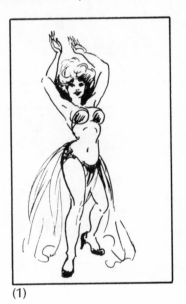 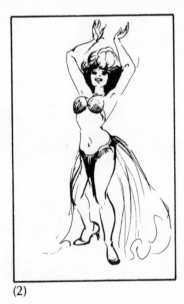

(1)   (2)

Belly Dance Basic Step

Back Bend and Arch (standing)

- Assume correct posture.
- Stand straight, feet slightly apart, left foot in front of right foot.
- Hands out at sides.
- Slowly lower your head backwards.
- Do not move the lower part of your body.
- Shoulders and torso follow head backwards until you form an arch.
- Lift head up, then shoulders followed by torso back up to original position.
- Repeat 3 times.

Do this exercise very slowly so that you get the full benefit from it. Do not strain yourself. Each time you do this exercise, lower your head and torso a little more. After months of practice it is conceivable that you could do a complete back bend all the way to the floor.

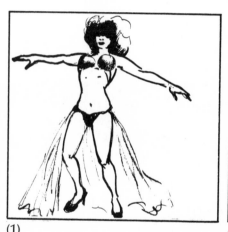 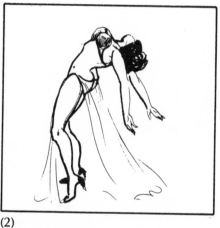

(1)   (2)

Back Bend and Arch (Standing)

CHANGING YOUR EATING PATTERNS

If you are more than a little overweight, you will need to do more than the exercises. Even professional belly dancers must watch their eating habits. It's easy to put on pounds and inches even if you are belly dancing every night of the week if you gorge yourself with the wrong kinds of food as soon as you get off the stage. I know. I have had personal experience with this problem, and so have many of my colleagues. It is not by accident that they have good slim figures.

The answer is, therefore, very simple. We belly dance as much as we can and we also follow fairly strict eating patterns. Notice I didn't use the word "diet." That word, I feel, has been belabored to death so I use a less imposing and oppressive term to which most women can relate without getting "uptight." Anyway, dieting is nothing more than a healthy eating pattern.

In this book you will be hearing about some healthier eating habits as well as belly dancing as an exciting form of exercise that will burn up some of the calories that can so rapidly add weight.

For many people, altering eating and exercise patterns is a chore that it is not easy to cope with. I am no different, and it is a "must" for me to watch my food intake because I am so often in the public eye. In my profession, bulges are desirable but they must be in the right places!

Even though you are not a professional dancer, you know that excess weight can handicap your career and your social life. You are, in a sense, "on stage" too, because people you meet every day judge you largely by your appearance. Your local city is your stage—your world is your stage—on which you want to look your best. Welcome to the club.

Besides the question of appearance, you know that keeping physically fit and at the proper weight can be important to your health. What you eat and how much you eat means a great deal to you.

HOW SEVERAL WOMEN HANDLED
THEIR WEIGHT PROBLEMS

Norma T. is a very close family friend of mine who followed poor eating habits for many years. I'm glad I was finally able to persuade Norma to change her eating patterns, because she was ruining her health with what she ate. Here is a typical day of Norma's meals:

Breakfast 1 quick cup of coffee with 3 heaping teaspoons of white sugar
1 prune danish or some other such pastry

Lunch 2 slices of pizza
1 large coke
1 candy bar

Dinner   2 hamburgers, complete with rolls
              1 cup of corn
              1 portion of french fries
              1 dish of chocolate ice cream

As you can see, these meals consisted of mostly starchy, fattening, non-nutritious foods. I won't even comment on her "in-between-meals" snacks or the two or more drinks she felt she had to have before she went to bed. At every meal, Norma wasn't happy unless everything was piled high on her plate. The result of these eating habits was an accumulation of about fifty pounds of excess flab. Norma did not look well or feel well.

Norma and I often talked about proper eating patterns, and I soon realized her philosophy and mine were on a collision course. She wanted to *enjoy* her life and eat what made her feel good. Finally she realized that she wasn't doing herself or her body any favors by stuffing herself with a pile of trash, and at last I even got her to the point where her eating patterns fell into line with my ideas of nutrition. Nowadays, she will not touch any of those fad foods. Here is a typical day for her now:

Breakfast   ½ grapefruit
              1 cup tea with honey
              1 slice whole-wheat bread
              1 egg

Lunch   avocado, watercress and shrimp surprise stuffed in pita bread
              1 cup fresh fruit salad
              1 glass milk

Dinner   1 cup soup
              meat balls kebab
              1 cup brown rice pilaf
              1 cup beets
              fried eggplant covered with plain yogurt
              1 cup tomato and cucumber salad

Norma's goal now is to have a balanced eating pattern every day of her life. Your goal should be likewise. Try to eat meals similar in proportions and nutritive value. Of course Norma is much happier with this approach to eating, and needless to say, she really looks good these days. She has lost the fifty pounds and is now maintaining her present weight beautifully. No more "pizza stomach bulge" for her. She has also become more aware of the benefits of exercise, and she is doing belly dance exercises religiously. I gave her a copy of them about a year ago.

Over the years countless women have come to me for advice on weight problems, figure problems, and related personal problems, and I have dealt with their problems in my own way. In many cases I have urged them to try belly dancing exercises and improved eating patterns. I think they are finally realizing that, through belly dancing, they can find a key to many of their problems. Take Joanna M. for example. She was an acquaintance of mine who had been putting on some pounds. It was about a year after she gave birth to her second child, and she was still about twenty-five pounds overweight. I was belly dancing at one of the resort hotels in the Pocono Mountains in Pennsylvania, and she had come up for the weekend. We started to talk about exercise and she casually asked me what I did to keep in shape. I gave her a couple of simple belly dance exercises, but I also told her to cook a few of my Middle Eastern recipes, which I later sent to her. I met her again a couple of months later and she told me that, after nearly three weeks of practicing at home to music while taking care of her baby, she found herself with new energy and her musical exercise period became the part of the day she looked forward to the most. She became so interested that she asked me for some more movements, exercises, and recipes, and she is now a very proficient Middle Eastern dance afficionado. She tells me her sex life has improved one-thousand percent, that she is twenty-five pounds lighter, and that she is loving every minute of her new-found body.

Then there was Lillian T., who was uncertain about what was causing her husband to "stray." She had been married only seven years and could not understand why she and her husband were having so many arguments over the most petty things. We had long discussions about that, and we decided that she was probably not paying enough attention to the way she looked and he was noticing it. I could see that she thought my life was most exciting and that she hoped to get some hints from me as to how I managed to stay trim and full of life. Of course I gave her my whole philosophy on eating patterns and proper exercises. I also gave her an autographed picture of myself in all my glory. This picture encouraged her to lose some weight, and she told me that after she lost the weight she made a belly dance costume for herself. Then she posed in costume and took some pictures of herself, some of which she hung in the bedroom. Her husband thought this was a splendid idea. He been showing her picture all over town. Somehow that experience, and my advice, motivated her to start eating sensible meals (she loved my yogurt recipes) and to start doing many of my exercises. Well, Lillian is still happily married to the same man.

Norma, Joanna, and Lillian are only a few of the many women who have been helped by my advice on healthy eating and by my belly dance exercises.

"TUNING IN" ON A NEW LIVING CHANNEL

Being fat does not necessarily mean being unattractive, since many people carry their fat well. Medical doctors, however, have told us that there are definite health problems associated with being overweight, and that unneeded weight will greatly decrease your life span. Some of you may feel your life span is long enough for you, considering the miserable shape our world is in today. Sometimes long life hardly seems worthwhile, does it? But for most of you, those who would like to stick around a little longer and live a more healthy, productive life, I have a whole new "channel" for you to tune into. This channel will give you good exercise tips and valuable nutritional fun recipes. After you get all that material together, I'll tell you how to throw a Middle Eastern party to celebrate your new-found life!

THE MIDDLE EASTERN WORLD

Let me now give you a little background on the art that is the basis for these exciting dance exercises. As I explained earlier, the term "belly dance" originated from *belledi dance*, "belledi" being an Arabic word meaning village or country. When it travelled to America, "belledi" turned into "belly" dance, perhaps because the French called it "danse du ventre" or dance of the belly. It has also been called "nautch dance," nautch deriving from an Indian word "natya" which means dance. The term "hootchy-kootchy" has also been used to describe the dance, but where this originated is anybody's guess. One thing is certain and that is that it is more than a *belly* dance because every part of the body is used in the dance. The most correct term to use when describing the dance is "danse orientale" or "Oriental dance" (raqs al sharqi in Arabic). The dictionary describes the belly dance as an Oriental solo dance, performed by a woman, emphasizing exaggerated movements of the abdominal muscles. Today the French and Arabs use the term "Oriental dance" (danse orientale) to describe the belly dance. Therefore I will refer to the belly dance as the Oriental dance from now on in my book.

When I first heard the term "Oriental dance" I immediately associated it with the Far East, such as China. However, I have become more educated about the origins of the term and feel more comfortable with it now. You see, the word oriental also means "of the East" or "Eastern," and since the dance came from East of the Arab countries, the Arabs called it the danse orientale or "dance of the East."

LIVING YOUR LIFE WITH ZEST

My book is dedicated to the love of life and the joy of being. I hope that through it you too will develop the zest with which I live my life. Here is to stimulating exercises and proper eating habits that will ultimately result in healthier bodies. We all have within us the essence of beauty. It is up to each one of us to nurture it and cultivate it into reality.

Through my Oriental dance exercises and diet I am going to help you achieve a trim and healthy body. One of the great side benefits of this whole program is that it will open up a whole new culture to you. It will help you to get out and meet new friends and start a whole new life. Through the Oriental dance you will build a bridge to another world.

If you've ever been to a Greek, Turkish or Middle Eastern wedding and the band strikes up a çifte telli (an Oriental dance tune), you'll see even the very old people out on the floor, and indeed you will see the very young imitating their elders. Children start at a very early age and go on until they too watch their children and grandchildren do this dance.

In many of the dance studios today you not only see young, shapely women learning the dance; the majority of participants are middle-aged ladies seeking a new lease on life. Some studios even have classes for grandmothers. This dance knows no limits as to age or sex, and that's the great thing about it. The older folks leave their classes feeling revigorated, not with aches and pains. If you feel any aches at all, you will feel them only the first couple of times after your rusty body embarks on this program. You're going to feel better and better each time you do these exercises and start on a nutritional eating program. Give it a chance and it will lead you to great things.

For example, my program helped Larry M. find a gorgeous wife. Larry was a 250 pound heavyweight. He was definitely not happy with this weight because on his 5′ 6″ frame the extra pounds did not look good. This overweight detracted from his attractiveness. Together, we decided that he needed to lose at least 44 pounds. With my help and lots of nutritious yogurt for snacks he did this in only six weeks—a little faster than I would have recommended. Once in awhile he would cheat a little; however, as the weeks went by he got better at watching his food intake. He got married soon after he lost all this weight. His wife is a great help to him because, out of sheer coincidence, she happens to be an Oriental dancer. Guess what? She's teaching him to do the Oriental dance, and I hear that he is getting to be so good that he may join her act.

HOW TO GET STARTED

In keeping with the spirit with which this book is written, namely to open up your mind and body to a healthy, new, exotic and exciting world, there are a few things that I would like you to start doing in order to get into this spirit.

1. Visit your local Oriental dance studio and ask to be put on their mailing list for their shows and other activities.
2. Visit your local Greek, Turkish, or Middle Eastern nightclub and drink in the atmosphere created there.
3. Visit your local Greek, Turkish, or Middle Eastern restaurant and start sampling the foods.
4. Visit your local public library and read up on the Greeks, Turks, and Middle Eastern peoples.
5. Visit your local Greek, Turkish, or Middle Eastern tourist office and get some posters and literature about that part of the world.
6. Visit your local Greek, Turkish, or Middle Eastern food stores and browse around.
7. Start thinking Oriental dance.
8. Start analyzing your eating patterns very carefully.
9. Start treating your body well by giving it proper exercise and rest.

Continue your exercises on a regular basis and you will derive the following benefits:

1. You are going to enjoy them beyond belief.
2. They will mold your body into the kind of shape that you can be proud of.

3. They will give you a control and coordination of your body that you never thought possible.
4. They will give you a self-confidence that will lead you to new and exciting things.
5. They will help you to become a more sensuous person.
6. They will help you build stamina.
7. They will help you to become more graceful.
8. The sky's the limit with the Oriental dance.

DIETING WITHOUT A DAILY MEAL PLAN

You will be able to lose up to four pounds a week if you faithfully follow my program. This is a slower form of weight loss than the usual crash diets because I want you to achieve a new life style that will be beneficial to you for a very long time.

No attempt has been made to give you a daily meal plan. I get terribly bored with a diet when I have to eat this or that on a Monday, a Tuesday, but never on a Sunday! Instead, you choose your own pattern. These recipes can be used in any eating pattern that isn't boring. I find that I can eat almost anything without gaining weight if I control the portions I eat and of course get the proper exercise. One word of advice—never go back for seconds, especially if you are trying to lose weight rather than just maintaining your present weight.

You do not have to take a calorie counter around with you in order to lose weight. One of the reasons I developed this eating pattern is the very fact that everyone was becoming too calorie conscious. It's so much easier just to cut down on your food intake rather than trying to remember how many calories of this or that you can eat.

May I again urge you to eat well-balanced meals. Remember the basic food groups are: milk or milk products; meat, poultry, and fish; vegetables and fruits; whole-grain or enriched breads or cereals; some oils and fats. A balanced meal would therefore include something from each of these basic groups. If you make sure that you eat something from each of these food groups every day you will be well on your way to making your body the healthy temple it should be.

YOUR "NORMAL" WEIGHT

Most people reach their normal weight between the ages of twenty and twenty-five. With each added year, fewer calories are needed to maintain this normal weight. However, people from their thirties on usually eat as much as they did early in life and therefore become physically less active and store their excess calories as fat.

Studies have shown that the average man who lives to be 65 weighs what he weighed between the ages of 18 and 24. The average man who lives to be 75 weighs 8% less than he did between the ages of 18 and 24. Women who live to be 65 can be 6% heavier than they were when they were between the ages of 18 and 24. People run serious risks if they carry around extra weight. From these statistics you can see that your chances of living longer are increased if you keep away excess weight.

There is no "quick way" to reduce that is safe and lasting and brings long-term results. Weight control requires a healthy balance between food intake and physical exertion on a steady basis. I am not extolling an extreme reducing diet because, even though these diets are successful in bringing your weight down, they do not help you to develop an eating pattern that *keeps* your weight under control.

Before starting any weight reduction program ask your doctor to advise you. Remember, each person is an individual and for that reason what is good for one may not be good for the other.

SOME EATING TIPS

I am going to list here some general tips I think are essential in providing a more nutritious eating pattern and ultimately a healthier you.

1. Consult your physician periodically for medical advice.
2. Remember that nutritive elements, vitamins, and minerals are necessary for a healthy body.
3. Eat foods that will give you the required level of protein, minerals, vitamins, and other nutrients.
4. Watch out for foods containing high cholesterol levels (saturated fat). Use polyunsaturated oil, such as safflower, corn, soybean, sunflower, and sesame. Polyunsaturated fats help the body to get rid of newly formed cholesterol deposits in the arterial walls. Medical research has shown that too many fatty foods can be damaging to the heart and blood vessel system. Trim off visible fat from meats before cooking and choose lean cuts of meat.
5. Most of all control your food intake.
6. Avoid excess salt in your diet. I see many positive steps being taken by food manufacturers in this direction lately. A

major producer of baby foods has eliminated salt from its products and has also reduced the sugar content.

7. Use recommended cooking methods for meat, fish, and poultry: baking, braising, roasting, and sautéing. Proper handling of your food will help preserve the nutrients in it. Do not overcook your food.

8. Under no circumstances use refined sugar. The refining process removes the nutrients.

9. Use natural foods such as unpolished whole brown rice which has vitamin B1, and beet or cane sugar which has natural minerals.

10. Avoid packaged popcorn, potato chips, and french fried potatoes.

11. Exercise in *moderation*. This is a key word on the road to good health. For example, carbohydrates in large quantities can only put on extra pounds. Most nutritionists will agree that some carbohydrate is necessary each day in order to maintain good health; however, be sensible about the amount you take in.

Most diseases can be traced to the lack of proper nutrition and proper exercise. No group of medical people will deny this fact; it has been proven over and over. For example, a research team has been very successful in getting people to cut down the risk of heart attacks. They suggest simply that you stop smoking, lose weight, and eat foods with less cholesterol and saturated fat. "Right on," researchers!

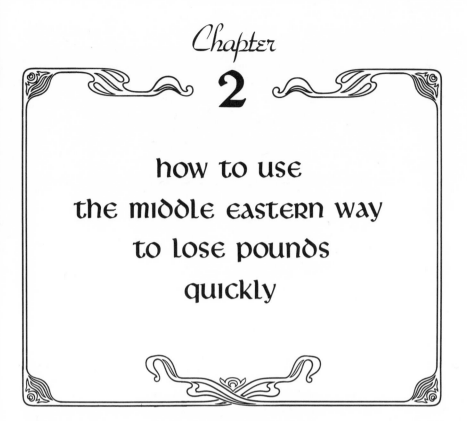

Chapter 2

how to use the middle eastern way to lose pounds quickly

WELL-BALANCED MEALS

The recipes in this book will allow you to achieve a varied eating pattern. Though I do not give you a specific menu for each day of the week, I would like to give you eight examples of well-balanced daily menus with a Middle Eastern, Greek, and Turkish touch. These will act as a guide to the kind of balanced nutritional menus you should be preparing. Please note that a helping should never be more than one level cup.

Breakfast	1 cup assorted fruit	1 cup fruit
	½ cup cottage cheese	1 egg (onion eggs, scrambled)
	1 tablespoon wheat germ	1 glass skim milk
Lunch	1 4 oz. glass tomato juice	1 cup tea (hot or cold)
	½ cup Greek salad	1 avocado pita
	4 asparagus spears	1 cup jello
	1 slice whole-wheat bread	

Dinner	1 cup egg and lemon soup	1 cup clear soup
	1 helping lamb brains	1 helping meat and okra
	½ cup eggplant salad	4 sprigs watercress
	½ cup carrot plaki	2 slices tomato
		½ cup ambrosia dessert à la Joan

Breakfast	1 cup grapefruit sections	1 glass unsweetened orange juice
	1 slice feta cheese	1 banana
	4 black olives	¼ cup soy nuts
	1 cup Turkish coffee	
Lunch	1 glass unsweetened apple juice	1 glass skim milk
	1 eggplant pita	1 health salad pita
	½ cup romaine lettuce salad	1 helping yogurt and fruit gel
Dinner	1 helping baked bluefish	1 cup clear chicken soup
	1 helping spinach pie	1 helping roast chicken with pine nut and currant stuffing
	½ cup cauliflower salad	½ cup green beans with olive oil
	½ cup sliced beets	1 slice boiled pumpkin
	1 slice honeyed melon	½ cup tomato and cucumber salad, 2 lettuce leaves

---

Breakfast	½ grapefruit	1 glass grapefruit drink
	¼ cup dates	1 egg (spinach eggs)
	1 peach, pitted and sliced	
	1 tablespoon wheat germ	
Lunch	1 asparagus pita	1 raw beef pattie
	1 glass borani cocktail	1 cup Greek salad
		1 glass yogurt fruit drink
Dinner	1 cup yogurt soup	1 helping yogurt kebab
	3 stuffed grape leaves	½ cup grated cabbage
	2 stalks steamed broccoli	2 slices fried eggplant
	1 stalk celery (chopped)	½ cup beet salad
	½ cup pearl onions	

Breakfast	½ canteloupe	1 8 oz. cup plain yogurt
	½ cup brown rice (cover	½ cup assorted fruits
	with plain yogurt, optional)	1 tablespoon raisins
Lunch	1 cup spinach and egg salad	1 cup fresh vegetable soup
	with yogurt	1 slice buttered whole-wheat toast
	1 glass vegetable juice	
Dinner	1 helping calf's liver	1 skewer swordfish kebab
	½ cup tomato and onion salad	4 boiled okras
	1 helping zucchini salad	½ cup steamed spinach
	½ cup steamed spinach	1 small steamed turnip
		½ grapefruit with 1 spoon honey

USING YOUR SENSES TO LOSE WEIGHT

These menus will mean absolutely nothing to you if you don't do some analyzing of the "behind-the-scenes" things that affect your daily life. For example, you are blessed with five glorious senses: hearing, sight, smell, taste, and touch. You use them every day without so much as a second thought. I want you to become very much aware of them and to use them in an ordinary everyday way that will benefit you. Then I want you to take them a step further and add a little Middle Eastern spice to them and use them in an even more heightened manner.

Hearing

You hear that voice within you saying that you are eating too much. Listen to it. Do not listen to the voice that says, "Eat some more of this lovely chocolate-covered cake." Listen to the voice that asks, "Is this good for my body?" Listen to the voice that says, "It's time to do your exercises so that your body will be healthy and beautiful." Listen to the lovely crunch of fresh wholesome vegetables, fruits, etc., not to the ugly crunch of biting down on a sugar-filled candy bar.

Listen to the tempo of your body. Is it going in a bright, healthy, happy way, or is it dragging in a sluggish, tired manner? Your eating and exercise pattern can help it run well. Proper food and nourishment will help your body wind up and run normally.

Sight

Your sight is bombarded with numerous enticingly packaged "poisons." Close your eyes to them. For example, the beautiful, sparkling white, bleached-to-death rice looks clean and wholesome. The brown rice may look dirty and unappetizing, but it is far more nutritious. Open your eyes to the nutritious products in your local food stores.

Look at yourself in the mirror. Do you like what you see there? If you don't, you must cut down on your food intake and you must exercise to create that image that you would prefer to see in that mirror.

Smell

You smell freshly brewed coffee and you go ape over it. You can't wait to devour a cup of it. But, is it good for you? Is the caffein content going to add any healthy nutrients to your system? Don't let your sense of smell run away with you. Learn to smell the healthy qualities in foods. Ignore the smell of unhealthy foods such as hot dogs. Instead, smell the success you are going to have with your new eating pattern and exercise program.

Taste

Your taste buds are the "naughtiest" and most troublesome part of your body. They lead you into the darkest alleys to eat some of the most unhealthy foods imaginable. Learn to control them. This will probably be one of the most difficult senses to control, so do it gradually. You can be pretty cagey when you want to be, can't you? Well, be cagey with your taste buds. Give them a little of what they want mixed with something that they are not too crazy about. For example, cut up some lovely fresh strawberries and dunk them in that unflavored yogurt. Add less and less fruit each time, and before you know it, down will go that unflavored yogurt all by its lonesome self.

Educate your taste buds so that they will appreciate the healthy, unprocessed, fresh food products. You are probably saying to yourself, "Oh, my taste buds aren't going to listen to me." Wrong, they will. They will give in to you if you are persistent and firm with them.

Touch

This is my favorite. Touch yourself. Go ahead. Do you like what you feel there? No? Well you can do something about that. Watch your food intake carefully, do your exercises faithfully, and you will come to enjoy touching those newly acquired lovely curves of yours. No one enjoys touching flabby, "yucky" flesh.

FOCUSING ON YOURSELF

Now that you have been slightly awakened to a few of the things that you can do with your senses, I want you to go on to some of the positive benefits that can be culled directly from the Oriental dance world. In order to do this I would like you to titillate your senses with the whole being of the dance. The dance did not appear in or from a vacuum, so to benefit thoroughly from the aura of it, I am going to ask you to heighten your five senses—hearing, sight, smell, taste, and touch—further by immersing yourself into things that are Middle Eastern.

You perceive stimuli coming from within your body and from outside your body. The foods you eat stimulate your body in one way or another. Through proper eating with a Middle Eastern flavor, I am going to give you a set of tools to stimulate your body in a way that I believe will be beneficial to you.

Your body, through the senses of hearing, sight, smell, taste, and touch, grows and develops through those stimuli it receives. I am asking you to stimulate your body with the danse orientale, and through it enhance your whole well-being with the culture from which it evolved.

Your feelings of perception are heightened when your organs of sense are fed the proper stimuli. So now let me show you how you can develop your senses through the danse orientale. First, let us take your sense of hearing. Have you ever really listened to the vibrations of your world? Stop for a minute and just listen to the sounds around you. We in the modern world especially are constantly bombarded by sounds—the sirens of the ambulance, police cars, or fire trucks, digging in the streets, jet planes flying overhead, subway trains, and so on. But then there are sounds closer to your being—your heart beat, oh how it races after you have run up a flight of stairs; your nostrils emit an ever-so-soft, soothing sound which gets louder when your nasal passages are blocked or when you take a deep breath. How nice to hear the sound of your breath. Without it there would be no life.

SOUNDS OF THE MIDDLE EAST

Is all this focusing on something? Yes, because from now on I want you to become more aware of the sounds around you. Turn up your volume, so to speak, on your hearing tube and listen, listen, listen. Before you even start your Oriental dance exercises I want you to start listening to the sounds of the Middle East, Turkey, and Greece. Visit a Middle Eastern nightclub, start listening to the music, to the voices of the singers as they wail out their tales of woe, of tears and depression, of love and of happiness. Listen to the couple talking next to you. Maybe you will be lucky and get someone talking the foreign tongue of a faraway land. Listen and hear the music and the foreign sounds beckoning you to distant shores. Listen, really hear and enjoy the sound vibrations.

You can hear the sounds of the Middle East and Greece on the streets of New York. You can go to the streets in Astoria, Queens, close your eyes, listen, and if you did not know that you were in New York you could very easily believe that you were in Athens, Greece. Walk down Atlantic Avenue near Court Street in Brooklyn, and—voilá!—there you are in Syria or Egypt or some other place in the Middle East. New York City is a very cosmopolitan city, and one takes those sounds for granted. Listen in your city and see whether you can find the sounds of the Middle East, Greece, and Turkey. Of course if you can afford it, travel to the Middle East, and there you can obtain the truly deep immersion into the culture.

SIGHTS OF THE MIDDLE EAST

How poor you would be culturally if you could not see, if your eyes were closeted in darkness. Thank God that you have your eyesight and can glorify your body by seeking out the sights that will give you pleasure. The danse orientale is a pleasurable sight to behold. You watch a good professional dancer going through her routine and you cannot help but stimulate your sense of sight. Your eyes will be dancing fast as she spins and whirls around the room, then they will calm down as the slow undulating movements of her chifte telli or taksim hypnotize you. Then all of a sudden she will wake you up as she concludes her routine all aburst with an intense, bright rhythmic pattern.

The dancing will bring sparkle to your eyes and so will the food of the Middle East. The kitchen is stocked full of beautiful, nutritious foods to stimulate your eyes. Feast your eyes on them.

SCENTS OF THE MIDDLE EAST

The smells of the Middle East can be exciting and different, as indeed any country other than your own can be. We will forget about the camels here folks! Enhance your appreciation of the Middle Eastern culture by taking in the aroma of its vast kitchen. Visit a nearby restaurant, and before you eat the food, let the steam from your plate float up to your nostrils and then really inhale the spices that will come at you in a very subtle way. Middle Easterners use spices in their food but they do it in a delicate way. It is unlike Indian cooking with its hot curries or Mexican food with its hot chili sauces. Typical Middle Eastern spices include allspice, anise, basil, cinnamon, coriander, cumin, dill, garlic, marjoram, mint, parsley, rose water, saffron, sage, sesame seed, thyme, and tumeric. Not a bad list, eh?

The exotic perfumes of the Middle East are also haunting smells. Jasmine, roses, frankincense, and myrrh are used for incense and perfumes. The incense of the Middle East can take hold of your mind, and—poof!—in a cloud of smoke you are whisked away on Ali Baba's magic carpet up into the clouds. The air in Morocco is often filled with the smell of the genus *heliotropium*, especially a plant called arborescens which has small, fragrant purple flowers. Every seasonal river valley of the Middle East is sweet with the fragrance of mimosa and oleander.

TASTES OF THE MIDDLE EAST

Then we come to those taste buds that give us all so much trouble. Oh do we love to taste sweet, fattening things in our mouths. The Middle East is no different with its display of baklava, etc. If you have never tasted some of the pastries, then you should do so just to try them, but then forget about them, I find that nutritionally, the amount of sugar used is very detrimental to your health. If you do need something sweet, stick to the pastries made with honey. Actually, you could substitute honey for sugar in your recipes, but I personally do not eat any of those sweet desserts because I do not believe that they will serve my body well. I do not believe that they will serve your body well either. I would rather you satisfied your taste buds eating foods that will nourish your body. In Chapter 11 I have included some very nourishing dishes with a Middle Eastern flavor to them. Get out to the ethnic restaurants and see how the experts do it. Look, taste, eat, and learn.

TOUCHES OF THE MIDDLE EAST

To heighten your sense of touch, go out and start touching things. In the Middle East, even the men like to touch each other. Men touch each other when they dance and when they greet each other. This is not a sissy act; it is a warm, friendly gesture equally enjoyed by both men and women. You are happy to see someone, why not embrace? But no, in many cultures male children are taught at an early age to suppress their feelings. Even female children sometimes get this same limitation put on them. I say no, do it the Middle Eastern way—greet your friends warmly with a handshake, a kiss and a hug, all three.

Do not be afraid to touch others and even yourself. You would be amazed to find out how easy it is to find out where your extra lumps are. One great place that lumps like to live and flourish is right around your waist. Have you ever noticed that? It's up to you to evict those lumps and let them stay away forever.

For many years I taught art, and one of the projects I always made the children do was to make a "feely" box. In a shoe box they would place all sorts of things with different textures. A hole would be cut in the box where they could put their hands into it. They would exchange boxes with each other and have to guess the materials of which the things were made. I did this with the children because I wanted them to start touching things and really get into the different types of surfaces things have.

DEVELOPING YOUR "SEVENTH SENSE"

All of one's senses should be developed to their utmost, and through the Middle Eastern culture I would like you to develop a kind of seventh sense. People speak of a sixth sense when one is able to know how things are going to turn out before they actually happen or if one has a certain heightened feeling about something. Well, I would like you to go beyond that and develop a *seventh sense*—that of being able to live your life to its fullest in a most healthy, sensible, and loving way. So read on and start developing that seventh sense. If you work on all your senses and color them with the Middle Eastern touch, and if you follow my advice on eating sensibly and exercising faithfully, you will lose your extra pounds with steady, constant application of my suggestions.

Jonelle S. is a sensitive human being who lives her life using her "seventh" sense. She lost 21 pounds in 7 weeks on my eating plan and exercise program. She now weighs 120 well-distributed pounds. Men are flocking to her beautiful, healthy body and her charming sensitive ways. Though this weight loss took place 3 years ago, she is maintaining her new weight without any difficulty. That "seventh" sense does help, and you too can develop it.

Here in America many people look upon an Oriental dancer as nothing more than a gorgeous piece of flesh—a hunk of meat. I must agree with them in one respect in that most Oriental dancers do have gorgeous bodies. But that's where I draw the line. Oriental dancing is an art like any other dance form and should be treated as such. Many dancers have had a very difficult time bringing this point across to the general public. We are constantly struggling to keep the dance on a high level and to take it out of the gutter where so many have kept it because they saw a profit in so doing. Those people are the "meat merchants" who would do anything to make a dollar.

Before you embark upon preserving your body the Middle Eastern way, using Oriental dancing and good eating habits, I want you to become aware of why you are going to embark upon this approach. Why don't you take a quick look inside your mind and body? I am not suggesting that you just look at yourself in the mirror and explore your contours. That may be helpful to give you an idea of how much weight you have to lose and to start a love affair with yourself, but you have to go beyond that.

Your personal doctor can help you with this task. He can help you to become familiar with the inner workings of your body. That is where your outer beauty comes from. Doctors never seem to give out health and nutritional information without your prodding them, so it's up to you to find out the limits of your body. Your doctor can analyze you and help you search out your deficiencies, but it's up to you to carry on from there in developing your "seventh sense."

CHANGING BAD HABITS

There are certain facts with which you should become familiar in order to have general good health and to keep that heart healthy. Some things are hereditary and you have no control over them. You cannot change your genetic makeup. But you have a whole set of things over which you do have a great deal of control. For example, you can control your smoking habits. No one has to smoke, and the sooner you give it up the better off you'll be for it. I do not smoke, but I gave myself the smoke test just to check out the information that the American Cancer Society has been providing about the dangers of smoking. Before several of my performances I smoked a few cigarettes just to see what effect they would have on me. The effects were disastrous. After my show I experienced shortness of breath and a generally queasy feeling. Result—no more smoking for me.

Another thing that you have control over is the amount of fatty substances you eat. You should eliminate most of the fatty foods from your diet. Is your heart ever going to thank you for that! Too many fatty foods in your diet can lead to heart attacks.

You also have control over the amount of exercise you do each day. You should make exercise a regular part of your daily routine. If you want to go by numbers, it is necessary for you to burn up 3,500 calories more than you consume in order to lose one pound of fat. I go by my "seventh sense" and exercise regularly without counting anything.

Have you ever thought about what makes you tick? Wouldn't you like to be built of the stuff that those well-advertised wristwatches are made of? Think of all the abuse you could take and still come out of it ticking! Since we weren't built of the same stuff as those watches, and since we can't get too many spare parts for our precious bodies, we just have to take the best possible care of them that we possibly can. We can train our bodies to work like a precision instrument.

Like a car engine or any precision machine that must be kept in top condition in order for it to run efficiently, the body has to be kept in top shape in order to keep it going efficiently. Your body, the highest precision instrument in existence today, has to be strong enough to work under the most adverse conditions to ward off a million and one things such as drugs, disease, pesticides, tobacco, and pollution of every sort. It is important for you to find out as much as you can about how your own body functions, and I am sure that you will gain an increased respect and admiration for it.

Everything you do in life relates to your physical and mental well-being. If you abuse your body by getting small amounts of sleep, poor nutrition and no mental exercise, the precision instrument that is your body will soon wear out. Its parts will wear out before you know it.

GETTING ENOUGH SLEEP

Get enough sleep and rest. Notice I am not telling you the number of hours you should sleep, because each of us is different and our sleep requirements vary. Some people function fine on four hours sleep, some need as much as nine hours sleep to get through a day. If you feel sluggish when you awaken, try getting more sleep the following couple of nights. If you feel better, then you don't need an expert to tell you that that's the amount of sleep you should get each night. If you don't feel better, increase the amount of sleep for a couple more hours until you find the amount that your precious body needs. A sluggish feeling can be attributed to many things, but if this feeling occurs when you awaken in the mornings, try the above plan.

For heaven's sake don't depend on artificial ways to make you sleep. If you have problems sleeping, a good idea would be to do some exercises just before you retire. They will relax you to a point where your body will welcome the idea of sleep. Also try eating a cup of yogurt at that time; it will help calm your stomach. Conversely if you need an "eye opener" in the morning, do your exercises then. Whatever you do, regulate your sleeping pattern so that you go to bed at approximately the same time every night.

BUILDING A HEALTHY MIND

Have you ever given thought to what goes on in your mind? If not, how about starting now. A healthy mind does not just come out of space. Like anything else, you should nurture it. You should feed your mind healthy "foods" just as you feed your body healthy foods. I have not yet come up with a complete set of exercises for your mind, but I have included a couple of exercises in this chapter for you, and I can give you some helpful ideas to help you further. First of all, don't develop a one-track mind. If all you can think about is growing peaches in your garden then your garden will never be enriched to include some new and exciting varieties of fruits or vegetables. If you think creatively you can develop a fascinating garden filled with exciting things. Maybe if you gave it enough thought you could develop a process for cross-breeding peaches and pears to develop a new fruit. You don't want to remain stagnant.

The idea is to keep your mind in constant flux. Sitting in front of the television all day and night is not only unhealthy for your body, but it is also unhealthy for your mind. Your mind should be constantly stimulated. I am not saying that you shouldn't watch TV, but I am saying that you should exercise your mind in other ways too. In the Middle East people are still talking to each other. In our country it seems that the television set has replaced that lovely way to discover each other's ideas and feelings. Try alternating your TV viewing with other activities. Enroll in a class. Take up needlework, join a health spa, join a book club, start Oriental dance lessons. In other words, stimulate your mind to new heights with new ideas.

Begin your mental exercises with some quiet meditation. This can help you physically as well as mentally. As you sit quietly and meditate for any length of time you will reduce your blood pressure and slow your heart beat. Now you can begin your mental exercises.

One fun exercise I do for the mind is the following:

- Sit down in a quiet corner away from everyone.
- Bend your head and hold it in both hands.
- Clear your mind of all thoughts.
- Think about a faraway place like Greece.
- Then think about another country.
- Continue to change from country to country.
- Come back to America and reality.
- Continue for about ten minutes.

You don't have to get an expensive plane ticket to travel around the world. You can substitute various themes for your mind expansion; e.g., you can imagine yourself in many different professions, different people, different animals, different flowers. The possibilities are endless, and you will have a lot of fun and your mind will be stimulated.

All this will lead to mental alertness, which should be one of your goals along with healthy exercise and eating patterns. Any exercise you do causes chemical changes in the brain, and this will alter your thinking considerably. When you are physically fit you also tend to be mentally fit because exercise acts as a protective device against emotional stress. You build up a reserve of adrenalin which helps you overcome tension. This way your mind will be running on a number of different tracks to health.

A DAY OF EXERCISING AND EATING CORRECTLY

The expensive way to lose pounds the Middle Eastern way would be to sign up for classes at your nearest Oriental dance studio. However, since most of your budgets are limited I am going to list what a typical day of exercising and eating correctly should entail.

This was the plan that Jane T. followed with great success. She is a court stenographer whose only exercise at work is walking in and out of the courtroom. After the first 3 weeks on my dance and diet program she lost 12 pounds. She had to lose 30 more pounds but did this at a much slower pace—15 weeks. After the initial weight loss she said that she had gotten lazy at times but was able to bring herself back to doing things right.

In Chapter 7 I have detailed the Oriental dance exercises for each part of the body for your further perusal. More low-calorie recipes can be found in the chapter with low-calorie recipes of exotic Middle Eastern dishes.

So many of the food staples of the Middle East are full of the nutriments needed in your system that you can hardly avoid staying healthy if you vary your Middle Eastern dishes. You don't need to take vitamin and mineral supplements because as far as I am concerned they are an expensive and unnecessary entity if you eat the proper foods. Take lamb, for instance. It is eaten extensively in Greece, Turkey, and the Middle East, and it is filled with vitamin B and protein and has less cholesterol than most other red meats so popular in the American diet. Listed below are some of the food products used in the Middle East, Greece, and Turkey giving their nutritive value to further illustrate my point:

1. Apricots —laetrile (vitamin B_{17})
2. Apricots, dried —iron, minerals, protein, vitamin A
3. Black currants —bioflavonoids
4. Eggplant —calcium, iron, magnesium, phosphorus, potassium
5. Figs, raw —calcium, pantothenic acid, phosphorus, potassium, protein, vitamin A
6. Fish —This is full of vitamin B_1 (thiamine), vitamin B_{12} (cobalamin). The prophet

Mohammed thought that sea water was pure and therefore said it was okay for one to eat the animals that live there. Fish also has high-grade protein, copper, iodine, iron, polyunsaturated fatty acids, potassium, zinc, sulphur, phosphorus.

7. Grapes —calcium, phosphorus, potassium, vitamin C

8. Green beans —calcium, chlorine, magnesium, phosphorus, potassium, vitamin A, C

9. Green peppers —vitamin A, C, phosphorus, potassium, magnesium

10. Nuts —proteins, unsaturated fats, B-complex vitamins, vitamin E, calcium, copper, iron, magnesium, phosphorus, potassium

11. Okra —calcium, magnesium, phosphorus, potassium, vitamin A, C

12. Parsley —Here in America we use this product to decorate our food. Fresh parsley is very good for you because it contains vitamin A, C, iron, protein, potassium, calcium, phosphorus

13. Pistachio nuts —protein, potassium, calcium, phosphorus, vitamin A

14. Raisins —copper, vitamin A, biotin, calcium, magnesium, phosphorus, potassium, sodium

15. Sesame seeds —Particularly high in calcium, B-complex vitamins, A, D, E, phosphorus, iron, fluorine, zinc, iodine, potassium, magnesium, unsaturated fatty acids

16. Spinach —calcium, phosphorus, potassium, sodium, vitamin A, C, choline

17. Sunflower seeds—particularly high in protein, B-complex, A, D, E, F, calcium, phosphorus, iron, fluorine, zinc, iodine, potassium, magnesium, unsaturated fatty acids

18. Tomatoes —vitamin C

19. Yogurt —B-complex vitamins, vitamin A, D, protein, para-aminobenzoic acid

Here now is a typical day as a guide for you. If you follow some semblance of this routine over a period of six weeks you're going to feel and look like a new person. The times I give here can be changed if so desired. If your day begins at noon, carry on from there. Here I am starting at the time when most people start their day. The night before you follow this particular meal plan prepare your shish kebab so that it will be ready for the following day.

6:30 a.m.	That darn alarm goes off and you hit the snooze button to get 10 more minutes of heavenly sleep.
6:40 a.m.	Roll out of bed.
6:45 a.m.	Get your tape recorder or record player ready and put on your music. This will soothe your mind while you are getting up.
6:50 a.m.	Get your eyes open with a glorious cold water face wash and clean your teeth.
7:00 a.m.	Get into your exercise clothes or come as you are.
7:10 a.m.	Do exercises illustrated in this chapter.
7:30 a.m.	Take a quick shower.
7:40 a.m.	Have breakfast.

½ grapefruit
a cup of Turkish coffee (recipe given in chapter 11)
1 slice buttered whole-wheat toast
1 slice (½" thick) Greek feta cheese

7:50 a.m.	Prepare some lunch.

chopped egg, lettuce and tomato
1 pita bread
fresh fruit salad

8:00 a.m.	Dress and get going.
9:00 a.m.	Work, work, work.
10:00 a.m.	Take a break. You deserve a break today! Have a 5 oz. container of yogurt (no artificial flavoring or preservatives added).
10:10 a.m.	Work, work, work.
12 noon	Lunch
	Take out your pita bread and stuff it with the prepared mix. If you go out to lunch have some chopped egg, lettuce, and tomato on whole-wheat toast, a glass of milk, and some fresh fruit salad.
	After lunch take a walk.
1:00 p.m.	Work, work, work.
6:00 p.m.	You're home at last. This is your time. If you have a family make that perfectly clear to them. Put on your most comfortable caftan or lounging robe, put on some Middle Eastern music and relax. Forget the office, school or wherever your work is. Think of the exotic Middle East, Greece, Turkey, or wherever.
7:00 p.m.	Prepare dinner.

	See recipes included in this chapter. Lots more are in the chapter with Middle Eastern recipes.
8:00 p.m.	Relax with your family over a leisurely meal.
9:00 p.m.	Visit friends, watch TV, fight with the kids and/or husband, take in a movie.
11:30 p.m.	Indulge in your favorite pastime.

Or, if you are trying to lose weight rather than maintain your present weight, do the body stretches and limbering up exercises given in Chapter 5 for 20 minutes. If you are on a maintaining routine, 10 minutes are enough. Then soak yourself in a luxurious Vita Bath (Badedas) or some other exotic bubble bath for at least 10 minutes. Then go to sleep and rest your tingling body. You may have some more yogurt before you go to sleep. This is very soothing to the stomach.

THE ROLE OF MUSIC

Middle Eastern music is an integral part of all my exercises because music helps to soothe your soul and, depending on the kind of music you listen to, it can also help you to relax. A peaceful and serene mood is very important to bring to your exercises. The music also helps to make your exercises fun and to set a beautiful mood for you.

At this point I would like you to invest in the following two Middle Eastern records to give you a further taste of the music of that region of the world. I have listed here the tunes that you should use from these records for the exercises given in this chapter.

1. *Middle Eastern Soul*—Bob Tashjian, Souren Baronian—Carlee Records

   Side 1—Makhmoor Aghchig
             Gleli Yebouy
   Side 2—Geozlerin

2. *Strictly Belly Dancing—Ya Habibi #2 Vol. 1*—Eddie "The Sheik" Kochak—Scepter Records

   Side A—Cleopatra
           Chifte Telle
   Side B—Chutak Melody
           Shifte Armany
           Oud Fantasy

ORIENTAL DANCE EXERCISES

Now that you're well on the way with your exercises, I would like you to increase the time allotted for them to 15 minutes per day. Do the same limbering up exercises that you started off with plus the mind and body preparedness exercises before you go into these new Oriental dance exercises.

Mind Preparedness—Inner Body Ripple

- Assume a horizontal position, back flat on floor, hands at sides, palms of hands face up, and feet about 12" apart, eyes closed.
- Relax all your muscles.
- Start with your head. Empty it of all negative thoughts. Replace them with peaceful thoughts. Let these thoughts propel the rest of your body starting with your head and moving down to the tips of your toes.
- Reverse the process. Send relaxing waves from the tip of your toes and work them up to the top of your head. Keep alternating this inner body ripple for about 2 minutes. Slowly rise to a standing position.

This mind preparedness exercise and the body preparedness exercise are used to get you into the proper mood for your Oriental dance exercises. They are not an actual part of the dance; however, sometimes during a performance I find my mind and my body wandering off into the serene feeling that these preparedness exercises achieve.

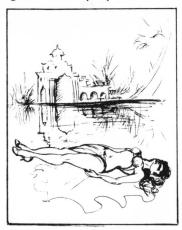

Mind Preparedness—Inner Body Ripple

Body Preparedness

- Assume correct posture, stand straight, hands at sides, feet slightly apart.
- Close your eyes.
- Try to picture a shangri-la, the most beautiful and serene place you can imagine. Imagine yourself to be the sexiest creature in this place.
- Tell yourself that you are the most beautiful person in the world.
- Relax your body.
- Tell yourself that you are going to nurture your body, you're going to develop the best body in the world.
- Relax and hold this position for about 2 minutes.

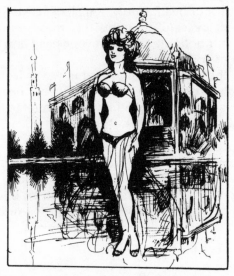

Body Preparedness

Head Slides

- Assume correct posture.
- Place both arms directly over your head.
- Place the palms of your hands together.
- Slide your head over to the inside of the left elbow.

- Hold for the count of 4.
- Return to the starting position.
- Slide your head over to the inside of the right elbow.
- Hold for the count of 4.
- Repeat on each side 5 times.
- Make sure that the rest of your body is perfectly still and that only your head moves from side to side.

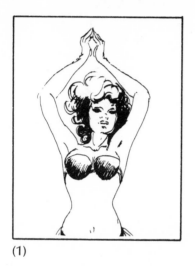

(1)

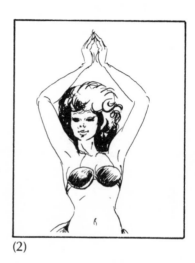

(2)

Head Slides

Slow Shoulder Thrusts or Pushes

- Assume correct posture.
- Hands down at your sides.
- Shoulders should be straight facing forward.
- Thrust left shoulder forward. Hold for count of 2.
- Return to starting position.
- Thrust right shoulder forward. Hold for count of 2.
- Return to starting position.
- Alternate shoulders and repeat 3 times.

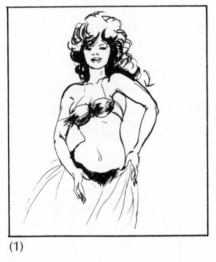

(1)

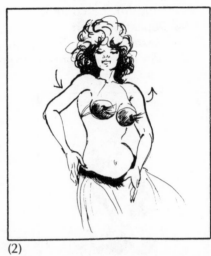

(2)

Slow Shoulder Thrusts or Pushes

Serpent Arms—Frontal

- Assume correct posture.
- Bring left arm up slowly in front of you.
- The shoulder should rise first, then the elbow. The forearm will follow, then the hands.
- Bend wrists and bring palms of hands up so that fingers point to the ceiling.
- Lower the left arm slowly, leading with the elbow.
- Repeat 3 times.
- Do the same with the right arm.
- Repeat 3 times.
- Then alternate arms. The left arm should be going up when the right arm is coming down.
- To achieve the snakelike effect make sure to lead with the elbows. The left elbow should be pointed towards the ceiling when the right elbow points toward the floor.
- The arms should pass each other about shoulder level.
- The arms should be curved and raised slowly and gracefully.
- Repeat 5 times.

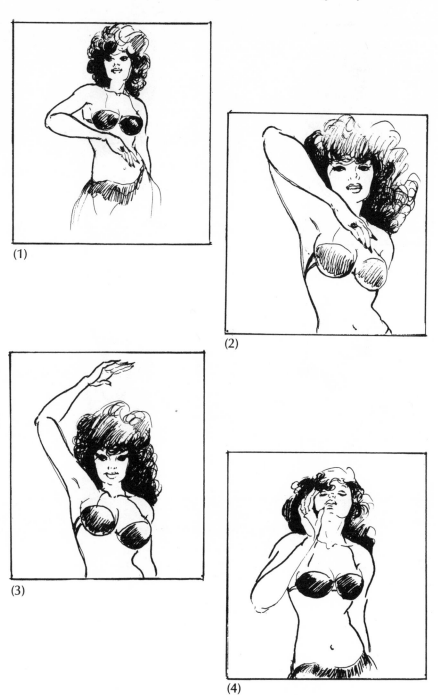

(1)

(2)

(3)

(4)

Serpent Arm—Frontal (Single)

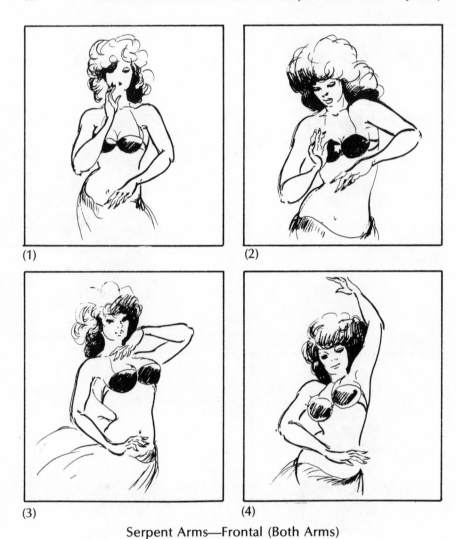

(1)   (2)

(3)   (4)

Serpent Arms—Frontal (Both Arms)

Rib Slides

- Assume correct posture.
- Raise arms above the head.
- Lower body should be perfectly still.
- Slide your rib cage from the waist over to the left.
- Hold for 2 counts.
- Return slowly to starting position.

- Slide rib cage over to the right side as far as possible.
- Hold for 2 counts.
- Return slowly to starting position.
- Alternate sides.
- Continue for about 2 minutes.

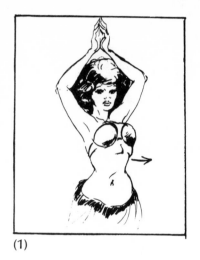

(1)

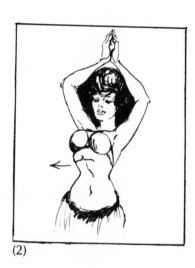

(2)

Rib Slides

MIDDLE EASTERN RECIPES

Included here are some nutritious Middle Eastern recipes to get you started on your new, exciting life style. These recipes are very easy to prepare and present a balanced meal. I have given you recipes for a complete dinner. Surprise yourself and that special person of yours with this mouthwatering treat.

Your responsibility to yourself at this point is to start controlling your food intake. Serve no more than a cup of each dish per person. Each person should have only 1 skewer of shish kebab.

Mint and Parsley Salad (Tabbouleh)

Arabic   serves 4 persons

1 cup fine bulghur (cracked wheat)
1 cup scallions or onions, finely chopped
½ cup mint, finely chopped
2 cups fresh parsley, finely chopped
2 medium tomatoes, finely chopped
1 cup lemon juice
¾ cup oil
salt and pepper to taste
a few large leaves of lettuce

_____

1. Soak bulghur in water for about an hour, then drain off all water.
2. Mix bulghur and scallions together thoroughly, add mint, parsley, oil, and lemon juice gradually and mix thoroughly.
3. Decorate with chopped tomatoes.
4. Serve, on lettuce leaves if you wish.

Lamb on Skewer (Shish Kebab)

Turkish and Greek   serves 4 persons

3 pounds lamb, cut in 2-inch cubes
1 cup red wine
⅓ cup oil
2 cloves garlic, crushed
3 bay leaves
1 teaspoon oregano
salt and pepper to taste
2 dozen mushroon caps
3 large tomatoes, sliced in quarters
3 green peppers, sliced in quarters
2 medium onions, quartered
2 medium eggplants, cut in 2-inch cubes

_____

1. Marinate lamb cubes overnight in mixture of wine, oil, garlic, bay leaves, oregano, salt, and pepper.
2. String meat on 12-inch skewers, alternating with mushrooms, tomato, green pepper, onion and eggplant.

3. Brush with marinating juices and broil on a charcoal grill or in an oven broiler for several minutes until the meat is brown.

This is a fun sort of dish and you can experiment with all sorts of variations. For example, try alternating lamb with only eggplant cubes, or only onions, or try other vegetables that I have not mentioned here.

Beet Salad (Pancar Salatasi)

Turkish   **serves 4 persons**

2 bunches fresh beets
3 teaspoons honey
salt to taste
2 quarts water
2 tablespoons oil
1 tablespoon vinegar
2 tablespoons lemon juice
¼ teaspoon garlic powder
2 scallions, finely chopped

---

1. Remove stems and roots from the beets. Scrape the beets lightly but leave the skin on.
2. Wash in cold water.
3. Put beets, honey, salt in a pot of cold water and bring to a boil.
4. Cook until beets are tender.
5. Cool beets and peel off the skin.
6. Slice beets very thin and place in a salad bowl.
7. Put beet juice in a small bowl and add oil, vinegar, lemon juice, and garlic. Mix well and pour over beets, cover and refrigerate.
8. Serve cold.

Vermicelli Pilaf (Sehriyeli Pilav)

Turkish   **serves 4 persons**

2 cups chicken or meat broth
½ cup fine vermicelli

4 tablespoons butter
1 cup rice (unbleached brown rice)
salt and pepper to taste

---

1. Boil broth until hot.
2. Sauté vermicelli in butter in a deep heavy saucepan until slightly brown.
3. Add broth, rice, salt and pepper.
4. Cover tightly and cook for approximately ½ hour until water is absorbed and rice is fluffy.
5. Serve hot.

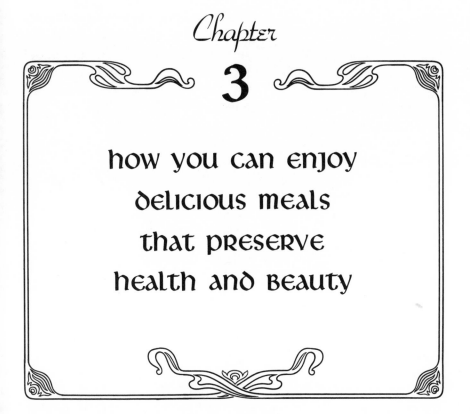

Chapter 3

how you can enjoy delicious meals that preserve health and beauty

To prepare delicious meals with a Middle Eastern, Turkish, and Greek touch you will need to do the following:

1. Gather an assortment of spices from that part of the world.
2. Accumulate various ethnic cookbooks. (I have given you several recipes to get you started.)
3. Purchase fresh food products from that part of the world. (A list of stores is provided in the appendix.)
4. Start dining out in some of the Middle Eastern, Greek, and Turkish restaurants around town so that you will become familiar with the foods.
5. Start thinking positively as to exactly what a delicious meal is. (For one thing, it does not have to be entrées of gooey stuff oozing with lots of fatty gravies, or desserts full of whipped cream and strawberry icing.)
6. Start developing healthy ideas of what you want your body to be.

Delicious meals do not have to be fattening. There are lots of tasty ways to prepare the same old foods to which you have become accustomed. My recipes will help you to do this. You can derive enjoyment from your delicious meals by:

—turning on to food of a different culture.

—preparing varied and interesting meals.

—eating nutritionally balanced meals.

—taking care of your body so that it shines like a beautiful eternal flame.

—eating more slowly so that your taste buds will be satisfied with less food.

—giving Middle Eastern parties (sans junk food) that will be the talk of the town.

—introducing other people to healthy eating patterns with a Middle Eastern touch.

Some people have the body metabolism that allows them to eat heaping mounds of all sorts of foods, do very little exercise, and never gain a pound. This is fine but I believe that sooner or later their bodies will holler for help and slow down to a sluggish crawl. Metabolic disorders cause all sorts of problems over which one may have no control. Your doctor could help you to sort them out and help you to correct them.

There are other people who fall into the other category of gaining weight as soon as they put the fork of food into their mouths. These are the people that I am trying to help the most because I know how frustrating this problem is for them. If I can help you to gain new confidence that will guide you through these difficult, frustrating days of your life, then I will have achieved my goal of helping you to have a more healthy and happy life.

Janice R. was one of these people who had this problem of gaining weight as soon as she put a fork to her mouth. She wanted to weigh about 128 pounds. I helped her achieve this goal over a period of 7 weeks. She weighed 150 lbs. before she started on my program. For her 5' 6" medium frame I recommended that she lose 25 pounds. She ended up losing 28 pounds which she hasn't gained back. A whole new world has been opened up to her.

REASONS YOU OVEREAT

There are several other reasons why one may eat too much. One is that there are certain ethnic groups where the mother literally stands over the children and stuffs food into them. You may belong to one of these groups, but more often than not you have all experienced this act when you go to a friend's house for dinner and you are asked by the mother if you would like some more rice pilav and you graciously decline, but before you know it the pilav is piled on your plate anyway. Sounds familiar? Certain groups make this their goal in life, so then you have this inbred in you from your childhood days and you continue the pattern in your later life. You perpetuate it and hand it down to your children, and so it goes from generation to generation. This tradition is dying out because many people are becoming more self-conscious about their eating patterns and are somehow getting around that persistent mother, great aunt, or whoever.

Another reason may be psychological. This is a very difficult problem to deal with because it may lie in a totally unsuspected area of one's psyche. If you can't pinpoint the psychological area that is causing you to overeat or if you can't do it by thrashing out your problem with a close friend, then I would certainly suggest that you seek professional help. I never liked to rush for professional help until I tried to help myself out of whatever rut I was in, because more times than not I was able to get out of situations without spending a dime.

This problem reminds me of a friend, Pat O., who had a definite weight problem and there was nothing that I or any of her other friends could do to get her to start eating sensibly and doing some exercise. We knew that her problem was not caused by heredity, a metabolic disorder, or any such thing because we saw that it went beyond any of these reasons. It seemed to us that something psychological was definitely causing her overeating. It was as if she was out to kill herself with food. There had been a few love problems, but we didn't think that they were anything special or out of the ordinary. (On this subject we were all experts!) Another friend suggested that she see her psychiatrist, and Pat tried that awhile. After a couple of months she came to me and asked whether I'd give her a few Oriental dance lessons. I was terribly busy at the time and couldn't give her private lessons, but I sent her to a friend of mine. I kept watching her progress and I started to give her my whole lecture about eating nutritionally and doing exercises on a regular basis. Well, I must tell you that Pat took up my whole "spiel" and today I consider her one of my success stories. She had to be helped to get herself together, to want to do something about her problem. There are many people out there who just need a sympathetic ear to help them on their way. Pat is looking great these days and besides that she has been bending our ears with the great insight she has gained into herself.

Social customs are another reason why people gain weight, get sick or otherwise abuse their bodies. There are some societies, for example, where heavy consumption of alcohol is a very definite way of life. It has been proved that liver diseases and other related disorders are high on the list of reasons for fatalities in these places. Here in America some of the customs of eating fast-food concoctions such as hot dogs, sodas, and other "junk" food cause all sorts of problems.

THE DANGER OF TOO MUCH MEAT

Another huge problem we have here is the high consumption of meat. This leads to heart attacks and other diseases. So many people are now paying for the so-called luxury item (meat) that is considered a sign of having made it and of being a success in our society. Fortunately, I have seen a great surge in the area of nutrition consciousness, and this can only lead to a more healthy society. Maybe we should thank God for the high meat prices because they have certainly curtailed the heavy consumption of meat. I am sure that you could add many other examples from your own experience where social customs dictate the intake of one product or another that could lead to all sorts of problems.

Heredity also plays a large part in your being the way you are. There isn't much you can do to change this, but you can learn how to enhance, nurture, and perhaps improve your God-given qualities. It is always good to learn about your background so that you can better deal with problems that may run in your family.

Other reasons for obesity may include thyroid deficiency, adrenal overactivity, or hypothalamic tumors.

Insurance companies aren't too thrilled with fat and obese policyholders, and for good reason. All studies indicate that if you carry around excess fat your chances of living a long life are shortened.

THE TROUBLE WITH "COUNTING CALORIES"

It is a simple fact that you become fat when you take more calories into your body than you burn up in your day-by-day activities. That is one of the reasons why I do not count calories even though caloric intake is geared to one's weight. I believe that since each person is a different human being it would be folly for me to tell you that you must have a caloric intake of so much and that you must do such and such amount of exercise.

Two Oriental dancers may have an entirely different life style, so it would be difficult to give one set formula for all to live by. Moreover, I find counting calories a definite bore. If you become aware, eat nutritionally, and do proper exercises you will lead a rewarding life without having to become a mathematician.

Other reasons for being overweight may include a low blood sugar problem, glandular imbalance, lack of exercise, eating too much of the wrong kinds of foods, and having an eating pattern that excludes vitamin-mineral supplements.

Now, what you have to do is isolate your problem and work on it. If it is a physiological problem you're going to need the help of your doctor. If it is a psychological one such as eating an overabundance of starches and sugars you are going to have to work things out yourself with my help.

SETTING REALISTIC GOALS

Throughout this book I will maintain that you do not have to set an impossible goal for yourself as far as your food intake goes. This goes for everything in life. It is most desirable to set goals, but try to set *realistic* ones so that you can have happiness and contentment when you achieve them. Setting impossible goals only leads to frustration, and this leads to stress which is the worst possible thing for your body. Indeed, you need to have goals in order to be motivated to new heights and to keep your adrenalin flowing.

Before you can decide on a goal it is important for you to understand what beauty, health, and nutrition mean because these things will become very important to you in your everyday life. If you concentrate on these things you will begin to feel a whole lot better about your life. The dictionary describes beauty, health, and nutrition in the following manner:

> *Beauty*—1. The quality that is present in a thing or person giving intense pleasure or deep satisfaction to the mind. It arises from sensory manifestations (as shape, color, sound, etc.) from a meaningful design or pattern, or from something else (as a personality in which high spiritual qualities are manifest). 2. an attractive, well-formed girl or woman.

Health—1. The general condition of the body or mind with reference to soundness and vigor: good health. 2. soundness of body or mind; freedom from disease or ailment.

Nutrition—the act or process of nourishing or being nourished.

With these definitions in mind, your goal should be to achieve everything that they speak of, because having the qualities of them is the ultimate goal to which you can aspire. You must strive for soundness of body and mind, to be an attractive, healthy person, and for an improvement of your psychological and physical well-being.

A SENSIBLE EATING PATTERN

The first thing you should do towards the goal of having a well-formed, sound body is to begin a sensible eating pattern. In order to do this you must begin to understand what causes you to eat yourself to death—and that is exactly what overeating does to the body—and then try to control the problem at its very roots. For example, if you've just stopped smoking and have now taken on the equally bad habit of munching chocolate bars, you have to recognize that this problem exists and should work on cutting down your consumption of them. You must bring yourself to the conscious awareness of what you are doing to your body and ultimately to your very life.

BOREDOM AND THE REFRIGERATOR

For the most part I have found that when I am bored and have nothing to do at home the refrigerator becomes a handy crutch, something to lean on to keep me from boredom. To prevent this from happening to you, you must find something for your idle hands and body to do. I love to paint and I am fortunate to have some talent in that direction, so I like to have a canvas available all the time. Painting is a great positive pastime, but if you don't paint, do something else that you enjoy: crocheting, knitting, reading, or even start writing your first book. This book kept me out of more refrigerators than I care to mention!

You can eat sensibly and lose weight. My research has shown that if you have a balanced eating pattern and embark on a programmed exercise regimen such as the one I have introduced here which is designed to produce physical fitness, you can control your weight. You just have to set your mind to it and take on a whole new attitude about your way of life. It will not be easy, but you can do it with the advice I have given you on your eating habits and exercise regime.

The nervous system coordinates all your body's activities in response to signals it gets from inside and outside your body. The brain of course is the big "director" or "conductor" of all the activities. There is a little section in your brain that causes all the problems many people have with eating. The brain, the most complex part of the body, is the organ that triggers hunger pangs after measuring the level of nutrients you have stored in your body. Oftentimes just the smell of one of your favorite foods is enough to start your salivary glands working, and bingo, you think that you are hungry and you go after that food with a vengeance. Your appetite is also dependent on the taste of the food, the appearance of the food, and your emotional state. Now if you can control these things through your brain waves, you've licked the problems of an over-active appetite. Of course if you can't, then you just have to start working on the problem in another way. If you could only find a way to control your brain in a scientific way then you'd have the whole key to controlling your food intake, and just think of it, you wouldn't have to worry about watching what you eat. I understand that delicate operations can be done to eliminate that particular section of the brain that causes all these problems. However, it is an extremely dangerous procedure and the risk involved is not worth it.

CONTROLLING YOUR BRAIN WAVES

What you have to do is to work on controlling your brain waves yourself. You are able to manipulate the signals that get to the brain. You are going to decide that you are going to control successfully the amount of food you eat. You are going to tell yourself constantly that you don't need all the junk food that you normally guzzle. You are going to help yourself achieve your goal. Once you have decided that you will start eating sensibly, you then have to work on keeping yourself convinced that this is the right thing to do. In time you won't have to work so hard at convincing yourself, it will be second nature to you.

No one should be allowed to put negative thoughts in your mind. If someone tries to discourage you, you will ignore them and their negativeness. If you try to find all sorts of reasons why you can't eat sensibly and control your food intake, then it's up to you to tell yourself in no uncertain terms that this careful study of your eating habits will make you a better person both physically and mentally. This kind of reasoning will ultimately make sense to you, just don't give up. It's going to be very easy, believe me.

HOW TO KICK THE "FAD-FOOD" HABIT

If you find difficulty kicking the fad-food habit all at once, then you will have to approach it with slow determination. Remember, you are in no hurry to fail. Take your time and you will succeed. Tell yourself that you will drop potato chips from your diet today. Next week you'll drop chocolate bars, and so on. I would recommend a quick, "cold turkey" withdrawal, but I'd like to give you the choice of the withdrawal suitable to your life style and to your capabilities. Under no circumstances do I want you to become frustrated with my program, because in addition to working on your physical well-being you are also working on your mental attitude, and you want to develop that into a positive one that will last a lifetime.

I use the term *withdrawal* because that is exactly what it will be for many of you. For example, I urge you in my book to cut out refined sugars completely, and to do so takes all the incentive you have. You should read labels on prepared food products very carefully. If a label lists sugar first it means that the product has more sugar than anything else. All you would be doing then is eating or drinking gobs of sugar. When I first cut refined sugar out of my food intake I had a very difficult time because I had to get used to a whole new taste pattern. This withdrawal is one of the hardest that I know. After awhile, with that control of your brain waves, you can do it and before long you will not miss the sugars at all.

You will also have to cut out all between-meals snacking, unless you are on a special diet for a particular ailment where you might have to eat about six times a day. Your body needs a regimented feeding pattern. Most Oriental dancers are on a late-night eating schedule, but they still eat at regular intervals unless they are still struggling to make a living! When they're having breakfast at 4 a.m. you're still sleeping. The idea is to keep the times you eat your meals consistent. I learned this the hard way. I used to eat at all different times of the day or night as the whim hit me. Not only that, but I used to "party" a lot and get irregular amounts of sleep.

HOW I RID MYSELF OF AN ULCER

All that, plus the stresses of teaching and of the world in general gave me a nice duodenal ulcer. Imagine an Oriental dancer with an ulcer? That was good for a few interesting conversations. I was under a doctor's care for awhile but that soon became a bore and I started to analyze my whole life style to see if I could help myself get rid of the ulcer once and for all. The ulcer diet was literally killing me. I could not stand all those insipid foods that I was told I had to eat to get well, so I started to experiment with various health food ideas and I started to watch my food intake very carefully. Some of the very foods that were "verboten" in my eating pattern had essential food nutrients that my body needed.

Finally I came to the conclusion that I could eat anything within reason and not have those awful pains I used to have. This is one of the reasons that I hate any kind of "diet." I hate to be restricted, especially to foods for which I have no desire. I was recently talking with a friend of mine whose husband has an ulcer and she said something which really made a lot of sense to me and sort of sums up my feelings about ulcers. She said, "Oh, it's not the food you eat, it's the mood you're in." My ulcers haven't bothered me for many years now, and my mood certainly has improved after I started eating foods I could enjoy. My doctor is amazed that I can survive all the great salads I eat.

A sensible eating pattern does not include overindulgence in alcoholic beverages because they destroy vitamins, especially vitamin B. Alcohol is a depressant which retards the metabolism or burning up of fatty acids in the blood. If the excess of fatty acids is not burned up, as I told you before, they form deposits on the walls of the arteries, the brain, or the heart, and that causes various diseases. There is nothing wrong with having a drink now and again, but do not make it a heavy daily habit. A little Turkish raki, which is a drink distilled from grapes, is a very soothing sort of drink and may be used for digestive purposes. You'll find that at many a Turkish dinner, which sometimes lasts for hours on end, raki is drunk all through the meal and no one ever gets inebriated. I guess that the congenial atmosphere and relaxed feeling help to bring about a calming effect on your digestive process.

The Middle Eastern kitchen is chock full of very healthy foods. Take for instance the okra (bamya). This vegetable has as much protein and nutritional value as soybeans which are an important source of protein. Bamya can be cooked until tender, allowed to cool, garnished with a little lemon juice and olive oil, and you have a refreshing vegetable dish. When it is cooked with chopped meat and a few spices it can become almost a meal in itself. The nutrition is all there.

Fiber is a very important part of one's eating pattern. It is found only in fruits, vegetables, and whole grains. The following items found in the Middle Eastern eating pattern are high in fiber content and should be included in your eating pattern: almonds, beans, chick peas, dates, dried apricots, dried figs, raw prunes, red and white currants, ripe olives, sesame seeds, and wheat.

Milk is my favorite drink with my meals. I once heard a famous nutritionist advise people to drink milk with their meals. He said that water, tea, and other beverages should be drunk about half an hour after your meals. I never did find out why he felt this way, but I respected his views so I have been following this pattern for a long time now and find it to be quite healthy. Somehow the milk settles my stomach. I also love to have a little wine with my meals now and again. I never drink sodas because of their sugar content and other artificial substances. Milk has not been a common drink in the Middle East because of lack of pasturization and other problems.

The Koran (Qur'an), which is the word of God and acts as a kind of guide to proper conduct by which the Muslims live their lives, tells us that one should eat and drink with gusto. It prohibits all liquor except when it is produced by means of honey, barley, wheat, or millet. If you are a good Muslim then you will live by this rule. I will go into the religion of Islam a little bit more later on.

WHAT TO DO ABOUT SECOND HELPINGS

Second helpings are a "no-no." If you ask for seconds, let's hope that you'll be like Oliver Twist and get slapped. When you catch yourself asking for seconds, talk yourself out of it. Remember your goal. No seconds, remember that. If you live alone, a good idea would be to buy small amounts of food that would, for example, last only a week. When you run out, that's it. You control yourself and never go running to the store to buy more food.

Half a grapefruit eaten before meals helps to depress your appetite. If you also get in the habit of eating it in the morning, that would be a good idea. It helps tremendously to ward off colds because of the vitamin C content. I have a gentleman friend who has eaten a grapefruit every morning for as many years as he cares to remember and he hasn't had a cold since he started this ritual. Another teacher friend had the same experience. The only difference was that she ate an orange every day before lunch. Her friend's mother lives in Florida and would send crates of fruit up to her daughter. She couldn't eat it all, so she would drag in an extra orange to school every day for her friend. Sometimes friends do come in handy. Citrus fruits should always be an integral part of your eating pattern. In the Middle East, Greece, and Turkey they have the greatest juicy and succulent citrus fruit.

Your stomach will "shrink" after awhile and you'll find that you won't crave food as you used to. It's all a matter of disciplining your body to exist on less. The quality of the food you put in your body should be of the highest nutritional value. Put less food in, but make the quality the best.

WHEN YOU SHOULD NOT EAT

Never eat while you are tired, worried, or agitated in any way. If you eat under these conditions they interfere with your digestion. There are some illnesses that can also influence proper digestion of foods. This is just another reason why you should work closely with your doctor or nutritionist.

Emotions and all sorts of mental activity also influence your digestion, and there are particular sections in the brain that control the consumption and use of food. That's why I recommend that you bring a peaceful mind to your mealtime, because if your emotions are erratic, your food will find an unsettled reception and this will ultimately affect your well-being. Would you believe that through your emotions the time that your stomach takes to empty can also be affected? This is a fact.

TREATING YOUR BODY WITH RESPECT

If you could learn to control your emotional state in addition to your brain waves then it is my opinion that you wouldn't need to worry about anything like dieting. All you would have to do is direct your brain to eat small, healthy portions of food. In lieu of this control it is most important that you treat your body with respect and protect it from everyday evils—poor exercise and abominable eating habits.

If you lack emotional control, then you require a somewhat structured regime to make up for your lack of control. It's almost like being in the Army—a soldier does not question his orders, he just carries them through. So you too must set certain goals for yourself and go straight ahead with their implementation, never stopping to question their validity. It is okay to question the validity of your goals before your commitment so that you can set proper goals for yourself, but never question them after you have made the commitment.

In summation then, what I am saying is that in lieu of being able to wish away your flabbiness, sluggishness, and creakiness it is necessary to give your body a constant physical, mental, and internal workout. Set some reasonable goals for yourself and then attack them with all you have got. Never look back for anything negative that will prevent you from reaching your goal.

STICKING TO THE "BASICS"

Remember, you must stay away from food fads and stick to the basics that have been around since Adam. Remember the problems he had with the apple? Well, it has been around ever since and I would consider it a basic. There has been a lot of controversy as to whether an apple a day does keep the doctor away. The way I look at it I feel that it will not hurt you to keep that ancient fruit, the apple, in your diet. Another basic is spinach. I wonder if they had spinach in Adam's day? If so, Adam could have been as strong as Popeye.

Basics, my dears, basics. The trouble with diet fads is that they place too much importance on one or two foods and throw all the others away. This kind of irresponsibility can lead to serious problems—to deficiency diseases and even to eventual death, believe it or not. What I am recommending is a back-to-basics approach to eating. In schools today that's all we hear—let's go back to basics. The sugar coating has to be taken off reading, writing, and arithmetic, and off of your *foods* so that you get the benefit of the simple things in life once again.

When I speak of "food fads" I refer not only to new artificial foods but to things like a diet that recommends that you chew your food 100 times before you swallow it, or to popping 150 vitamin tablets every day, or to a recommendation to eat beef on Monday, fish on Tuesday, fowl on Wednesday, but never on a Sunday. A balanced eating pattern is what your body responds to best and what your body needs.

Until now, as I said before, no one has found a way to completely control the brain, but you can achieve a limited amount of control if you assume the right attitude towards the food you put into your body. You should also practice your exercises daily.

YOUR NEW LIFE

You will soon see that your attitude towards life will change drastically. You will gain renewed energy to attack your daily life, which will become less tense and stress-ridden. You will increase your efficiency at home, on the job, and even when you play and relax.

Exercise strengthens the heart and increases the amount of oxygen that is carried through the body, and this provides more energy for the body and for you. Proper nutrition also provides more energy for the body. When increased oxygen gets to the brain it clears it up so that better thinking processes can take place. You are also going to work off your tension through routine exercises, and soon it will be "good-bye" to hypertension, headaches, and nervous stomach.

Motivation is the most important thing in changing your eating pattern. Many things can act as a motivation factor; for example, better health, improvement in appearance, impressing a new beau, or even getting back into a small-size dress you once filled out with fantastic, strategically placed curves. You must have a motivating factor going for you. Set a goal for yourself and do everything in your power to reach it. You are the only one who is going to be able to pull this off. You must also make up your mind that you are not going to fall back into unhealthy, slovenly eating patterns.

My friend Arlethia didn't fall back, and you should not either. Arlethia S. is a salesperson for a major department store. She was 50 miserable pounds overweight. As a result she couldn't take advantage of the great sales that her store ran. You ladies should know how difficult it is to get large sizes in a sale. Anyway, I met her in the store and saw her frequently on my visits there. I sold her on my approach to weight loss. She did my exercises religiously and became quite a Middle Eastern cook. Nine weeks later she lost 56 pounds. She took off the extra 6 pounds for luck. Today, she is doing fine and maintaining her size 12 figure. Her only complaint now is that she's spending too much money buying beautiful clothes.

I do not expect you to do Oriental dance exercises all your life, but I do expect you to make some form of exercise part of your daily life for the rest of your life. I also do not expect you to go through a starvation diet, become a size eight Miss World and then two weeks later slide back to an unsightly bulging bit of flab. The key, again, is to eat smaller portions of nutritional foods and gradually get rid of fancy "fake" foods such as frankfurters, pop corn, and potato chips.

Remember that hand in hand with any eating program you undertake, exercise is going to be right up there side by side with proper eating habits.

FIGURING YOUR PROPER WEIGHT

Before you start any exercise that will lead to weight reduction or stabilization it is important to find out what your correct weight should be for your particular height and bone structure. Correct weight depends on your age, sex, height, bone size, and muscular development. You can check with your family physician on what weight would be desirable for you. Insurance companies also provide this information.

When your body has an excess amount of fats it gets stored in fat cells as compounds called triglycerides. When your body needs energy it gets its fill from these storage areas. Of course when your intake exceeds your requirement you are in trouble. The fat cells build up under your skin, around your heart, kidneys, and other organs of the intestinal tract and just "hang out" there. This is the problem of which you should be thoroughly aware and should try to prevent as fervently as possible. Why do this to your body? It doesn't deserve this treatment. Be good to it.

I don't advocate counting calories because I think that it is an imposition to place on people. However, my philosophy follows closely the idea that one's calorie intake should be equal to calorie expenditure in order to maintain your weight if you think it is worth maintaining. If you are overweight then your calorie intake will have to be maintained at a low level in order to lose the desired weight. An alternative would be to double up on your exercises, but I believe in moderation and would not recommend that you spend an overabundance of time exercising. However, with less exercise your problems are bound to start when your calorie intake is always exceeding your expenditure of energy. This is when calories start being stored in your body in the form of body fat and you start seeing these unsightly bulges.

Proper eating and proper exercise go hand in hand. Your philosophy should be one of eating in order to stay alive. You are never to live to eat. This is always a dangerous route to follow. Eat to stay well, eat to be beautiful, and eat to survive. You should exercise to increase your stamina and endurance, to improve your muscle tone through your entire body, and generally to make you more limber all over.

AN IMPORTANT PRINCIPLE

An ounce of prevention is worth more than a pound of cure—a very good proverb to keep in mind throughout life. In other words, it's better to fence in the horse before he runs away. This principle, when applied to your life, can make for a healthier and happier life.

It would be careless of me to expose you to a way of life filled with healthy eating patterns and exercises without giving you some of my philosophy that led to these conclusions, if you can call eating patterns and exercises conclusions. For the time being I'd like to call them that.

The medical profession is here to stay, so why not participate in it to some extent. I believe that you have to treat your bodies like temples, and since the doctors of our modern society help build your bodily temples, it's a good idea to let them check your "building" from time to time. What I am talking about here is an approach to preventive health care.

Your physical condition can be controlled to some extent by your own personal wishes and desires. If you can control your psyche, you can control your physical well-being. Since few people have these powers, it is necessary that you make use of some preventive health care.

Everyone can have access to a physical checkup. If you don't have a private physician go to your friendly health clinic. Coupled with this idea is the business of good health habits such as rest and personal hygiene, good eating patterns, and proper exercise.

It's up to you to adapt proper healthful living to your needs. You are going to be the first one to know if you do not. Improper nutrition will get you if you do not eat the right foods. Did you know that if you lack certain nutrients in your diet this could prevent your blood from clotting and your wounds from healing? Lack of proper nutrition can make you feel listless, tired, and just plain "blah."

A PERSONAL BEAUTY SECRET

Your inner beauty will come from what you eat. That inner beauty is much more important than your outer beauty, because that is where it all starts. You cannot achieve an outer beauty if you neglect your inner beauty. Some women go around looking like a million dollars, but that million-dollar look comes from the million dollars of makeup that they have used to achieve the look. There is absolutely no point to looking well on the outside while your inside is crying for help. This way your body does not get the proper kind of treatment it deserves and must have in order to prevent an early decay that will eventually show on the outside.

It took me awhile to convince Mark Z. to eat nutritiously. He is a 6′ 1″ "fanatic" muscleman who is so into his body that he drives all his acquaintances crazy with his advice on how to improve their muscles and exercise their way to health. Surprisingly though he did nothing to control the quality of his food intake. The junk he ate was not to be believed. His body *looked* good on the outside, but I worried about his ultimate internal "breakdown." We discussed this and I convinced him to eat more nutritiously. Today he is so ecstatic with the way he feels that he's spreading the word about my program around his gym. He also told me that he lost 15 extra pounds (before he started my program he weighed 204 pounds) eating correctly. One year later he is still maintaining this weight loss and eating pattern with ease. Now all I have to do is to convince him to do some Oriental dance exercises!

You must develop a clean and healthy mind if you don't already have one. I don't mean that you're going to have to wash your minds out with soap and water à la teacher telling Johnny that she'll have to wash his mouth out with soap to get rid of the "filthy" words that spout forth from the little darling's lips. You are going to start thinking about your body in a more positive manner. You are going to have a love affair with your body. There is room in your heart to love yourself in addition to that other person in your life.

One harsh and realistic way to jog your mind into appreciating your own body would be to visit some hospitals where you see torn lives, bodies shrivelling up from disease and lack of care. Visit the slum of any city and you can see this very process in its early stages, before these people can't function anymore and either die or are admitted to a hospital in the hope that they will be put back together again.

Many of these problems stem from psychological beginnings, and these people have chosen to cop out of society and life itself. If these sights don't awaken you to the fact that you must take care of your mind and your body, I don't know what will.

If you don't need as strong an awakening as a visit to a hospital or the skid row of your city, then you must put some positive thoughts into your mind about your eating habits. Tell yourself that you are not going to go through life with one sickness after another and that you are not going to stay home night after night moping over a few extra pounds that are just hanging there.

SOME CHALLENGING QUESTIONS

I'd like to ask you a few questions to which your answer should be a resounding *no*. If you answer *yes*, then you must work on achieving a negative answer if you are going to succeed with my program. You will know that you're on the right track if your answers are already *no*.

Ask Yourself

1. Have other people been throwing little hints at me like, "Gee whiz, I remember when you were half the size you are now," or "We have room in our car but we need a thinner person."
2. Do I eat popcorn, chocolates, candies, and the like between meals?
3. Does my lunch or dinner consist of a fast hot dog at the corner stand?
4. Do I have french fries and other fried foods with almost every meal?
5. Is the only exercise I get walking from my easy chair to the TV set?
6. Have I been feeling sluggish lately?
7. Do I leave the dinner table feeling uncomfortably full?

I could go on with the questions, but I'm sure that you get the gist of what I am saying. You, and only you, can change the affirmative answers you may have given into negative ones. Then, and only then, will you be on the right track.

You are going to thrive if you give *yes* answers to the following questions:

1. Do I care how I look?
2. Have I received any compliments about my figure lately?
3. Do I eat at least one food product from each of the six essential categories of nutrients daily?
4. Do I exercise regularly?

5. Do I get all the sleep I need?
6. Am I stimulating my mind by showing interest in new things?
7. Am I relaxed doing my daily chores?
8. Do I have a new zest for life?
9. Do I want to have the allure and grace of an Oriental dancer?

The meals you eat can be prepared from the recipes I've given you. When you decide on the menu for the day make sure that you include foods from the six essential nutrients, namely, carbohydrates, fats or lipids, protein, minerals, vitamins, and water. Your food helpings should never be more than a level cup. Think cupful rather than bowlful.

Remember that you are not going to heap food on your plate. If the mound of rice you put on your plate looks like Mt. Everest, you are eating too much. One level cup of rice should be adequate for a meal. When you place the rice on your plate, flatten it out so it will look like more, and your eyes, and therefore your palate, will be satisfied. If you pile up your shish kebab to look like the height of the stones on the Wailing Wall in Jerusalem, you have too much on your plate. One skewer of most meat is enough protein for you at one meal.

The recipes I have included in Chapter 11 are some of the most delicious ones that I make. Many of them have a Middle Eastern, Greek, or Turkish origin and should serve to add a spark to your menus.

SERVING MEALS TASTEFULLY

When you serve your meals, serve them tastefully, even if you're the only one for whom you're preparing a meal. Add garnishing to your plate, such as a sprig of parsley, a couple of black olives, or a few slices of green pepper. One of my favorite garnishes is watercress. I love to eat it and it looks so pretty on the plate. I never quite knew what to do with the parsley that usually adorns my plate when I dine out at a restaurant. Someone once told me that parsley helps to take away the scent of garlic on the breath. It is important to satisfy your palate in an aesthetic manner. You're not serving slop to a pig, you are serving a sensitive human being—you and/or your family. You'll feel much better if you settle down to a beautifully served meal. Don't underestimate the aesthetics of the mealtime.

The atmosphere around mealtime should be conducive to relaxation. Some soft Middle Eastern music in the background while you eat your Middle Eastern meal will lend itself to providing the kind of atmosphere conducive to proper digestion. If the atmosphere surrounding your meal is one of confusion, your food will churn up in your insides, and before you know it, it's ulcer time and perhaps a number of other ailments. Your mind should be thinking pleasant things and your body should be relaxed. Put all your problems out of your mind. Relax, relax, relax, and enjoy. When was the last time you really enjoyed a meal thoroughly? Every day should be one of these days.

After your meal, before you or anyone else in your family do the dishes, give your food a chance to start on its journey through your digestive tract in the same peaceful manner. Have a couple ounces of Greek ouzo, Turkish raki, or Arabic arak to help you digest your meal. This is not necessary, but an occasional sip will help your digestive process. This can be taken in place of your coffee or in addition to it. Now get into your favorite easy chair, put your feet up, and relax for a while. But for heaven's sake don't lie down on the couch, your bed, or wherever your haven is.

THE ROLE OF FASTING

Fasting would be a great way to lose weight quickly. In most cultures that have fasting as a way of life it is never used for the purpose of losing weight. It is usually associated with the "cleansing" of poisonous substances from the body. Many people feel that this is a positive procedure since the body needs a "rest" from the usual food intake every so often.

We know that fasting was a way of life for many ancient civilizations, such as the Greeks, Arabs, and Romans. I personally do not like the idea of subjecting your body to sudden metabolic changes. I do not think that the body copes with this very well.

In the Middle East and Turkey they still go through periodic fasts, usually for religious purposes. During the month of Ramadan the Qur'an was sent down to be a guidance for the people. It asked people to observe an abstinence from all food and drink from dawn until sunset. It also asked them to keep away from their wives while going to the mosque. So you see this is not only a fast in terms of staying away from food, they also abstain from many other desires of the flesh, such as sex and entertainment.

Most of the people of the Middle East and Turkey are guided by the religion of Islam founded by the prophet Muhammad. For many, their religion is an integral part of their life. Through the holy Qur'an they get the word of Allah. A follower of Islam is called a *Muslim* (one who submits). There are over 50 million people speaking the Arabic language today, from Morocco to Indonesia, and there are at least 350 million people practicing the religion of Islam.

As in any religion, there are personal choices to be made. There is one Muslim group, the Khariji, who are extremely strict and forbid games, tobacco, music, and the like. This is one of the strong reasons for the late acceptance of the Oriental dance into the realm of respectability. Other sects are a bit more flexible and less strict, so you will see some form of the dance in many parts of the Middle East, thank goodness.

During a fast, the first couple of days you experience a bad taste in the mouth and/or a heavily coated tongue. Sometimes nausea, vomiting, dizziness, and other such things are experienced. I just hate the idea of having to experience all these uncomfortable changes within my body. For these reasons I am not recommending fasting as a regular way of life. A moderate fast of one day may be fine to flush out your system from time to time and prepare your body for the next couple of months of food intake.

Some people find fasting beneficial if they need to have rapid weight loss. I would suggest that if you are going to fast you check into a hospital where you could be constantly checked by a doctor. You must have professional help.

PRESERVING YOUR HEALTH AND BEAUTY

Your health and beauty will not come from sporadic fasting. It will come from an ongoing, concerted effort on your part to have only the best nutritional foods enter your system. You will preserve your health and beauty by:

—Cutting down your food intake.
—Cutting down on excess fats.
—Keeping the nutrients in your food by not overcooking it.
—Developing a sensible, nutritional eating pattern.
—Eating as many organically grown foods as possible.
—Imposing positive demands on your brain waves.
—Staying away from "junk" foods.
—Eating more organ meats.
—Avoiding between-meal snacks.

—Eliminating refined sugars.
—Eating in a completely calm atmosphere.
—Getting regular amounts of sleep.
—Avoiding alcoholic beverages.
—Doing regular exercises.
—Avoiding cigarettes.
—Getting regular checkups by your doctor.
—Slowing down your pace of life to avoid nervous disorders.

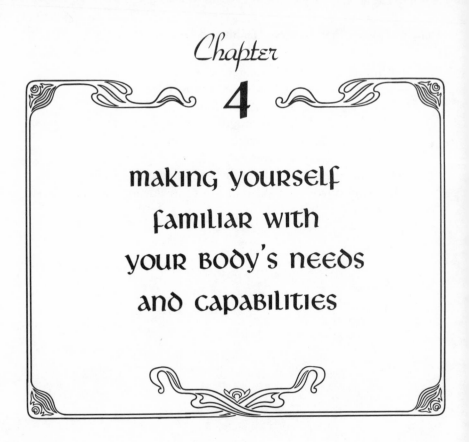

Chapter

4

making yourself familiar with your body's needs and capabilities

If you really want to start your new eating pattern and way of life in a scientific and precise way, you should go through some clinical tests and dietary evaluations. Some obvious nutritional defects that may go unnoticed by you can be easily observed by a trained person during a regular physical examination. Tissues such as the skin, hair, and teeth are examples of these easily observed parts of your body. It is most advisable that you see your personal physician for advice so that you can proceed sensibly on your way to good health. Keep in mind that your physical body depends upon your heredity, your environment, and your human experience for the shape and size it takes. For example, if your family tends to be big-boned, well-built people, chances are you will be too, and you could strive from now until eternity and you wouldn't become a svelte, petite person. What you should strive for is a way to enhance your own individual body structure.

DEVELOPING YOUR PARTICULAR BODY TYPE

There are over three billion people on the face of the earth and not one of them is exactly like another. Oriental dancers come in all different shapes and sizes and they all take care of themselves in their own unique ways. They all take very good care of their bodies. It's therefore up to you to develop your particular body type in your own way. Your bodily needs vary, and this is one of the reasons why each one of you has to do what's best for your own body. Each body should be treated as a unique entity. This is the chief reason that I have not given you a hard and fast eating pattern that schedules every morsel that you take into your mouth at a given time of the day. Besides, I find any kind of tight scheduling dull and very hard to maintain. I am sure that you know how difficult it is to stick to an eating pattern that is new to you. Moreover, the more radical the eating pattern, the more difficulty you will have with it. That is why most weight-reducing plans do not work for any length of time.

BALANCING YOUR EATING

Most people do not take the time or the money to evaluate their nutritional status. This I think is an error because it is very important for you to watch your nutritive intake carefully. If you cannot get to the doctor for this advice I will give you some help to put you on the right track. It doesn't take a doctorate to do something to help yourself. All you have to do is see that you have a well-balanced eating pattern. Eating patterns that are not well-balanced sooner or later cause problems. For example, if you were to be on a strict vegetarian diet you would be lacking in vitamin B_{12}. The thing to do under those circumstances would be to supplement your eating pattern with vitamin B_{12}. On a diet like this you would have to pay even closer attention to your nutrient intake so that, for example, you would get all the needed complete protein that you would normally get from animal-derived foods.

Actually it is very difficult even for a trained physician to accurately assess your nutritional status, but since he is a trained person he may be able to catch deficiencies that you may tend to overlook. You can be a very good judge of how your body is functioning. In order to do this you should try to learn what symptoms to look for and which ones keep cropping up and how to treat them. You can experiment very easily with vitamin and mineral supplements. What you do is take a vitamin for awhile and watch your body's reaction to it. If you break out in a terrible rash or some such noticeable difference in your appearance, you are obviously allergic to the vitamin or have no need for it, so you would therefore eliminate it from your shelf of vitamins. If you have no reaction to it, add another vitamin to your daily vitamin intake. Like anything else you do, do not go overboard with popping pills into your mouth, even though they may allegedly be "good" for you. If you use them as a food supplement rather than as the only source of nutrients, that's fine. Anyway you slice it, it is best to seek your doctor's professional advice before, during, and after you have superficially diagnosed your deficiencies.

I prefer to get most of my vitamins from natural sources rather than from a bottle, and I would urge you to do so too, even though this is very difficult nowadays because so many of the nutrients in our food are destroyed by food preservatives and harsh chemicals. It helps if you can grow your own food minus the chemical fertilizers, or if you can purchase your food from a reliable health food source. It is a pity that more constructive supervision by regulatory agencies isn't given to the foods you eat so that you wouldn't have to go out of your way to find "unpolluted" food products.

EXPERIMENTING WITH VEGETABLES

You can also experiment with vegetables and other food substances in this manner. I would never cut out all vegetables and concentrate on one; however, I would eat very large amounts of one particular vegetable and measure my reaction to it. This process of elimination is very similar to choosing your clothes. You wear one color and style of dress for awhile and then you find out that it's just not "you." The same thing happens with your foods. The way your body deals with foods is a fascinating process. I have noticed that at times my body cries out for certain foods; other times, when I suppose it has had its fill of that food, all of a sudden I don't want to see any of that particular food for a long, long time.

You may be asking yourself, "Why do I have to go through all this testing of my body's needs?" Well, at the base of all this is the word *nutrition*. I would like to describe nutrition as the science of giving the body nourishment. In other words it consists of the foods you eat and how your body uses them. We must remember that the relationship of humans to food is an important one, and a kind of relationship that you should constantly evaluate. You need the various nutrients in food to maintain growth and health. Am I eating the right foods? Do I need more vitamins, such as vitamin C or vitamin E? These are questions that you should be constantly asking yourself.

FOOD FOR YOUR BODY'S NEEDS

You should eat to satisfy your body's needs, not some need of your taste buds or your eyes. The former habit will build a truly beautiful body temple while the latter will destroy it. Your taste buds are very easily satisfied and should be watched very carefully. A great big strawberry shortcake with lots of whipped cream is a beautiful sight to behold; however, your body does not need it, only your eyes. Each of us needs nutrients but in varying amounts. It's up to you to find out exactly what your body needs.

Food goes through many processes in the body. These include digestion, absorption, and transportation of nutrients to various cells and their metabolism within them. The nutrients in food perform three roles in your bodies: regulating body processes, supplying energy and promoting growth, and repairing the body tissues. So isn't it important to feed the body well and give it the tools it needs to do these jobs properly?

In many cultures, food is used to conjure up magical powers and the like. In many societies today, food is no more than a matter of survival; fortunately for us in our supposedly more sophisticated society we are able to exercise some discrimination about the values of various foods. The kind of discrimination you exercise will depend upon you gaining important knowledge about the food you eat. You must therefore seek out this information from all the sources available to you.

Through science we have learned that nourishment of the cell is basic to the cells known as tissue, and this then nourishes the organs of the body, and finally the whole, very complex body. There are many other scientific data that you should investigate so that you will be able to deal with your needs in a more scientific way and therefore get better performance from your bodies.

THE PUZZLE OF PREGNANT WOMEN

You know the relationship between the quality of food a mother eats and the health of her offspring at birth. If a mother stuffs herself full of hard drugs while she is pregnant, her child will be born an addict. Studies have also been made as to the harmful effects that a mother who drinks heavily (more than two drinks a day) can have on her new-born baby.

Of course when you are pregnant your body is even more sensitive to things, and you have to think of that innocent little baby curled up in it. However, it always amazes me how careful most mothers are to take care of their eating patterns and other bodily functions during pregnancy. It is good that they are that concerned about their new offspring, but shouldn't they take the same care of themselves whether they are pregnant or not? Why the big fuss over the baby and not the mother too? These same mothers who pamper themselves for their babies over a nine-month period allow those same babies, when they are growing up, to eat all sorts of harmful candies and the like without so much as an attempt to regulate their junk food intake. Of course these mothers also go back to their old eating patterns, and proper nutrition goes out the window. All members of a family need nutritious food, not just unborn babies! I could cite numerous other cases to prove the importance of good nutrition for every member of your family, but I hope that I have proven my point with just these few.

Remember, the main purpose of food is to nourish the body. There are some secondary values that food fulfills, namely, the psychological value and the value of satiety. The important thing for you to remember is that you must choose your food wisely so that it provides all the nutrients essential to the proper functioning of your body. You must therefore keep in mind at all times the six main categories of nutrients—carbohydrates, fats or lipids, proteins, minerals, vitamins, and water—because you will have to see to it that your body gets its share of each of these on a daily basis.

The amount of essential nutrients that you need for normal bodily functions may vary according to your energy needs. Your needs depend greatly upon the type of job you hold and the daily functions you carry out.

THE CHANGES IN FOOD

When you eat food it must go through many changes to take a form in which it can travel to and be used by your cells. These changes take place mainly in the digestive tract of your body. This is only the beginning of a complicated process that serves to nourish your body. Therefore you must feed this complex organism—your body—the best possible foods that you can get hold of at all times.

Now, I would like to talk a little about the six categories of nutrients. Little did I know that I would have to be writing about nutrients at this point, or for that matter, at any point in my life. I remember sitting through nutrition courses in college being bored to death by all the technical information, but I am glad that I did and that I kept my notes so that now that I am more aware of my bodily needs I can utilize them and also share some of that knowledge with you. I will try to give you some understanding of these important facts that you should know, but I will keep them as simple as possible so that you will not be bored as I was. Maybe I should give my professor the benefit of the doubt here because there he was with about 36 hours to fill with information. For your part, you will be saved with this information because I want to fill only a small portion of my book with it.

KNOWING WHAT YOUR BODY NEEDS

Nutrition is an important study with which you should become familiar because it is so closely tied into your daily lives, and having an understanding of it can literally make the difference between life and death. Therefore, you must through even a perfunctory study make this study a priority so that you can know your body's capabilities and its needs. Later you can delve as deeply as you wish into this vast area of nutrition and bodily functions.

Carbohydrates

First let me talk a little about *carbohydrates*, which provide 50% to 60% of your energy. This is usually the largest single component in your diet. The carbohydrate is an energy-yielding nutrient. Carbohydrates provide the central nervous system with glucose (sugar) upon which it depends. We usually identify carbohydrates as starches and sugars. It is essential to the human nutrition because it helps in digestion and assimilation of the other nutrients. This is the one nutrient that gives you all the problems because the foods in this category are so good, and you should take particular care to regulate its intake very carefully, otherwise those bulges are going to begin to appear in the wrong places. The problem is that any carbohydrate that doesn't get used up in your body gets stored there in the form of fat. Somehow this is the nutrient you most abuse, the one with which you just keep stuffing yourselves. The reason you enjoy snacks chock full of carbohydrates is that they provide you with instant energy and your blood sugar level rises, but then your blood sugar level tends to drop very quickly, and before you know it, you start craving more cakes, sweets, and the like to get your energy up again. So you see, it's a vicious cycle. Therefore you must be on guard. On the other hand, when you do not have enough carbohydrates you start feeling sluggish, you lose your energy, and you start getting that old depressed feeling. Try to hit the happy medium by eating normal portions.

Carbohydrates are found almost exclusively in foods of plant origin. There hasn't been a dietary standard established for carbohydrates. Many diets that are lacking in carbohydrates are so bland it isn't even funny. That's why most people who go on them find it hard to stay on them for any length of time. Believe me, I am no different. That's why I tried to come up with an eating pattern that I, and ultimately you, can live with comfortably. Remember that the nutrients in carbohydrates are important to the normal function of the heart and brain, so you should not eliminate them completely as some diets recommend. Moderation would be the key here. Some very good sources of carbohydrates are fruits, grains, vegetables, and honey.

Fats

The next nutrient is fats or lipids, which provide 35% to 45% of your energy. This is the most concentrated energy-yielding group of nutrients. Fats are usually identified as saturated or unsaturated, depending on the degree of saturation of the fatty acids present. Did you know that fats contain over twice as many calories as carbohydrates and proteins? Some fat is desirable because, for example, deposits of fat beneath the skin serve as insulating material for the body, preventing it from being shocked when it gets too cold. The kidneys and heart are protected by fat deposits. Fat is helpful to you during an illness when you need increased energy. Fat helps to regulate the uptake and excretion of nutrients by cells. It also represents the chief form in which energy is stored in the body. The point you must keep in mind is not to build up an excess of fat, but to have some in your eating pattern. Since you do require fat in the diet, and it is a high source of energy as I said before, I would recommend that you watch the character of the fats you use. By that I mean instead of using fats of animal origin (high in saturated fatty acids), use fats of vegetable origin (high in monounsaturated and polyunsaturated fatty acids), such as safflower, peanut, soybean, sesame, and cottonseed, and use margarine instead of butter. These polyunsaturated fats help to keep your skin beautiful and, shall I use a pun and say, "oiled?"

Whole milk is a good source of these essential fatty acids. Some fat is needed in your eating pattern to carry essential fatty acids which are required for building such things as cell membranes. It is also needed to carry fat-soluble vitamins, A, D, E, and K. Since meat is a major source of fat in the American diet, it would behoove you to eat less of it. Too much meat (saturated animal fat) intake may help cause *arteriosclerosis*—one form of hardening of the arteries, a process which inhibits the flow of blood to your vital organs. And this may lead to strokes and heart attacks. There are a few exceptions to this rule: for example, fish and poultry contain highly unsaturated fatty acids and don't lead to such disasters as is possible with too much meat intake. I much prefer eating fish and poultry than heavy steaks. Somehow, my body doesn't get a heavy feeling from eating them.

If you include some fats like butter, whole milk, vegetables, and bread in your eating pattern you will be able to stand the idea of eating less. Have you ever tried to stick to a diet that had none of the aforementioned in it? Is it impossible to carry out for any length of time? What you have to do is gradually cut down your desire for food. Take it nice and slow and you will succeed. Fats and carbohydrates are two of the nutrients that muscles utilize and must have in order to be healthy. Some good sources of fats are whole milk and milk products, nuts, seeds, and vegetable oil.

Protein

Protein, which provides 10% to 15% of your energy is one of the most important nutrients. It is a component of every one of your living cells. If you don't have proper protein intake, your body cannot grow and ultimately neither can your body tissues. Protein is essential in the regulation of your body processes. You need protein to keep your brain, muscles, bones, skin, nails, hair, internal organs, and other tissues built up.

The value of this nutrient actually lies in its amino acid composition—the amino acids are the essential nutrients rather than the protein. Proteins are not stored in the body, and that is why it is important to keep replenishing this nutrient. You will find that if you do not have enough protein in your body your skin will stretch very easily and before you know it there it will be drooping all over the place. If you take a look in the mirror you can easily see whether you're getting enough protein. These flabby muscles are not only an external problem, they are also an internal one; for example, flabby muscles on the intestinal walls may cause malfunctioning there. You will also find that cuts and abrasions won't heal well.

A lot of foods that we normally call proteins would be more accurately described as *protein rich* foods. Their nutritive value is in the amino acid composition of their various proteins.

There is a difference in the quality of proteins. There are two categories of proteins—complete and incomplete. The complete protein or good-quality protein contains all essential amino acids in proportions capable of promoting growth. Complete proteins include soybeans, brewer's yeast, wheat germ, nuts, cottage cheese, American or Swiss cheese, milk, eggs, meat, fish, and fowl. The incomplete protein or poor-quality protein lacks one or more essential amino acids. The incomplete proteins include vegetables and fruits. You should therefore be careful to see that the incomplete protein is not the sole source of protein in your eating pattern, because when this deficiency exists no new tissue can be formed and worn-out tissue cannot be replaced.

I would say that about a third of your protein intake should come from animal sources of a high biological value. You should use the complete protein to supplement the incomplete protein, such as the use of milk with cereal, meat with rice, and so forth. You have to be careful with nuts because some contain complete proteins and others only have incomplete proteins.

Lack of protein in your eating pattern causes poor muscle tone and poor growth and tissue development. If your eating pattern lacks an adequate amount of proteins you may start feeling weak, you will lack vim and vigor, you will have poor stamina, and you will also have a low resistance to infection. An adequate level of protein intake is extremely important, especially when those stressful days appear. Then it would be a good idea to take in some extra protein to help rebuild your tissues that get worn out. Some good sources of protein include fish, meats, poultry, milk and milk products, eggs, whole grain, and soybeans.

Minerals

Minerals are found in your food and water. Fourteen of these are essential to an adequate eating pattern. The more important minerals are calcium and phosphorus, sodium and potassium, iodine, iron, and fluorine. Minerals are found in the blood, bones, muscles, soft tissue, teeth, and nerve cells. Minerals help to preserve the vigor of your heart, brain, muscles, and nervous system. They are also important in the production of hormones. Some good sources of some of the various minerals are:

> *calcium*—green leafy vegetables, shellfish, milk, and milk products
> *phosphorus*—poultry, fish, meat, eggs, legumes, nuts, milk, and milk products
> *sodium*—seafood, celery, table salt, milk products
> *potassium*—apricots, peaches, cantaloupe, watermelon, bananas, whole grains, dried fruits, vegetables (especially tomatoes, spinach and kale)
> *iodine*—table salt, sea salt, sea kelp
> *iron*—eggs, liver and other organ meats, poultry, fish, green leafy vegetables, dried fruits
> *fluorine*—seafood, tea, fluoridated water

Vitamins

Vitamins is a group of nutrients from which you need only small amounts. Scientists are still squabbling about the role of vitamins in our diet. We do know, however, that they aid your chemical processes by helping to convert food into energy and by regulating the manufacture of substances essential to the growth of your bodies.

We owe the name *vitamins* to Casimir Funk, a Polish scientist who discovered something he called "vitamine" in 1911. We have come to know this as "vitamins." I am confused as to the proper role of vitamins, as I am sure you are. One day you hear that you should have all the vitamin C your body can devour and then the next day you hear that it is harmful when taken in great quantities. Which of the researchers is right?

Another continuing controversy is the one over the benefit of vitamin E. It's hard for me to advise you when there is such a heated debate in all corners of the world. I would advise you to work on your vitamin intake with your personal physician. I personally try to derive most of my vitamins from fresh foods, with which this earth abounds at the moment. Of course if we continue to abuse the earth and its environs we may just have to rely on getting our nutrients from little capsules. It would be an interesting experiment to compare the functioning of two persons—one who ate only natural foods carefully prepared so that they would contain all the essential vitamins and other nutrients, and the other who got them in capsule form. So far I know of no such experiment being done.

There is no end to the list of vitamins. Some good sources of vitamins are:

Vitamin A—fish-liver oil, cream, lettuce, spinach and other green vegetables, cheese, carrots, apricots, eggs, butter, milk
B Vitamins—Brewer's yeast, whole-grain cereals, wheat germ, mutton, pork, beef liver, dark bread, cabbage, peas, beans, milk, eggs, cheese
Vitamin C—fresh fruits and vegetables, black currants, tomato juice
Vitamin D—fish-liver oil, cabbage, eggs, butter, milk, cream
Vitamin E—vegetable oils, soybeans, wheat-germ oil, raw seeds and nuts
Vitamin F—wheat germ, seeds, natural vegetable oils
Vitamin K—alfalfa, kelp, leafy green vegetables, green plants, yogurt, fish-liver oils, egg yolks, milk, polyunsaturated oils
Vitamin P—grapes, lemons, grapefruit, plums, black currants, cherries, apricots, blackberries
Vitamin T—egg yolks, sesame seeds
Vitamin U—cabbage, preferably raw

Water

Water is the most important nutrient going. Like most things one takes for granted, we hardly notice it at all. This is one nutrient that we can't live without for more than a few days. Water performs many roles in the body, such as a lubricant to help get food down your esophagus, as a catalyst, a body builder, a solvent for nutrients that must travel within the cells, and as a transporter of metabolic waste products. It is essential to absorption and circulation, it helps maintain normal body temperature, and it is necessary for all building functions of the body. I find it a great thing to reach for when I feel the need to munch on something, and as all good doctors tell you, you should try to drink at least eight glasses a day. Fruits and vegetables are a good source of chemically pure water. Lately I have been drinking a lot of bottled spring water and feel much safer doing so because recently there has been a great deal of talk about the tap water we drink. For one thing people think that there is too much chlorine in it. When I am feeling frugal, instead of buying bottled water, I boil tap water so that I can further purify it.

Water holds a very strong fascination for me, as you will see in Chapter 8. I love to drink it and I love to let it flow all over me. Maybe I should have been born a Pisces instead of a Capricorn.

A FLEXIBLE EATING PATTERN

The Oriental dancer's diet is one that you can carry out anywhere you go. You can find these foods in any restaurant in town. The specialty foods can be found in Middle Eastern, Greek, and Turkish restaurants, but many of the other foods are found in any store, and believe me I am not going to give you forty lashes if you go and eat Chinese food one day and Italian food the next. You have that leeway with my eating pattern.

In this day of the tight budget I haven't recommended too many high-priced foods. I love to eat a lot of health foods and I think they are very good to include in your eating pattern, but those prices are just unbelievable. It is my hope that one of these days you will be able to get wholesome foods for wholesome prices. Until then you will have to exercise wise and economical food budgeting and buying.

My eating pattern is not a monotonous one. How long can you eat fibers, cottage cheese, peaches and the like without going bananas? How many times have you gone on that cottage cheese and strawberries diet route and within a week, if that long, you are back to eating your basic meat and potatoes, and too much of them to boot? I went through long, tedious periods of the strawberries and sour cream eating pattern. I had strawberries coming through my ears. Then for a change I would throw in other fruits, but that became a bore after awhile also. I have seen hundreds of women go through this heartache of an eating pattern designed for quick weight loss, and within a very short while they go right back to eating tons of spaghetti and meatballs, chocolate cake, and so on. You don't need to eat cottage cheese and strawberries every day of your life to lose a few pounds.

What I am suggesting to you should be a very pleasant and easy way to lose weight (if that is your goal) or maintain weight if you already have a dashing figure. My idea will just tighten up things. It will also give you a pattern to follow for the rest of your life, and that is the kind of eating pattern with which you should be involved.

CONQUERING THE FADS

You must stay away from food fads. I keep stressing this because I think that it is one of the most important points I have to make, especially to the American woman. You must stay away from people who advocate miraculous properties in any one particular food substance and ignore all others. Some foods are worshiped in some cultures and scorned in others. Isn't this a little confusing? Some people say you should drink wine with your meals, some say drink water, some say drink nothing. Whom should you believe? My answer is, do what's best for you but keep it nutritionally sound. If you feel more comfortable drinking wine, drink it, but of course don't overdo it. One small glass with your meal should be sufficient. (Don't cheat and use your grandmother's one-gallon glass!) It will be up to you to differentiate between fact and fallacy in all the advertising with which you are bombarded. One thing I would recommend is that you stay away from carbonated artificial drinks. First of all you need a degree to decipher the artificial substances in them. What are phosphoric acid, sodium, saccharin, sodium citrate, and other substances going to do to your stomach? Of course the drinks are also filled with caffeine and artificial sweeteners. There goes heartburn number 50 in a bottle of carbonated beverage. Where are the nutrients? Another thing to stay away from is the hot dog, which is full of sodium nitrate.

Cholesterol is another subject of controversy, although most doctors agree that a small amount (150 mg.) is essential for normal bodily functions (one finds approximately 300 mg. in one egg). The problem with cholesterol is that if there is an excess of it in the blood stream, quantities become attached to the large and small arteries. Of course too much of this will block the arteries which could cause a heart attack, so it is important to watch your cholesterol intake carefully. This is one substance with which I exercise extreme caution.

Spices in Cooking

The Middle Eastern kitchen is full of variety. I can think of at least 50 ways that the Turks cook chopped meat. Compare that with the American one-track mind, wherein chopped meat means "hamburger." I love hamburgers, but how many times a week can you eat hamburgers without becoming fed up with them? (Maybe I shouldn't ask that question because I have a friend who could eat hamburgers every day of his life with no problem.)

Inevitably, when you become involved in the Oriental dance, whether or not your ancestors came from the Middle East, Greece, or Turkey, you inevitably start to savor the wonderful foods from that part of the world. Many of the staples are the same that you have in America and many other countries around the world. The spices used and the method of preparing them make the difference. So stock up on your spices now. Visit your local Middle Eastern food store and start sniffing the exotic aroma of spices into your system. It's amazing what a little bit of cumin can do for chopped meat.

Almost all of the Oriental dancers I've been in touch with use some of these spices in their cooking. Hummus and Baba Ghannouj and Greek salads are included in every Oriental dancer's eating pattern. The great thing about these and many of the other dishes that I have included in my book is that they are full of nutrients, and they are cheap and easy to prepare.

How Combining Nutrients Helps

Good nutrition is a way of life that you will have to acquire if you haven't already come to this realization. Nutrition can affect how you look by the influence it has on the various parts of your body and the characteristics which relate to your personality, and on your physical and mental efficiency.

There are lots of nutrients that have their own individual functions, but they still do not act independent of other nutrients. For example, vitamin E is more effective when taken with selenium. Iron is more effective when taken with vitamin C. It would be wise to check with your doctor on which ones act and work well together.

You must acquire good eating habits and good attitudes towards food in general. Moreover, you must assume responsibility for your own nutrition and of course if you have a family, for theirs as well. If you follow this path you will be able to prevent and treat many physiological conditions prevalent in our society today. You must therefore keep a check of your nutritional state by keeping a record of your body measurements, especially your weight and height, and a close check on your eating habits and patterns.

At this point I would like to recommend that you start keeping a record of the types of foods you eat and of the quantity you eat. If you do this and get some consistency into your life you will definitely be able to exercise the kind of controls that are needed to get that body of yours into excellent shape. At the end of each week you should go over your food intake and make sure that you are getting a balanced amount of nutrients so that you can have a healthy life.

Recording Your Food Intake

Just for fun, why don't you take this a step further? Before you change your eating pattern to a more healthy one, start recording your food intake. For one week before you start doing something about your eating habits, write everything down that you eat for breakfast, lunch, and dinner. Don't forget those in-between-meals snacks. Be sure to date this record. After you start getting more nutrition conscious, record your nutritional intake and compare the intake *before* and *after* you start following my advice. I am sure that you will notice a phenomenal difference. After several months, go back and look at that "before" chart again. It should give you quite a laugh at this point.

Your body needs nutritionally sound food. Respect your body and it will respect your wishes. A healthy body will serve you a long, long time. A sluggish, unhealthy body conks out at the first big traffic jam—a serious illness. With these points in mind, if you approach life in a positive manner your body will become a wholesome temple and your goals will be reached. You have heard the old saying, "You are what you eat." Well, I believe there is definite truth in this saying.

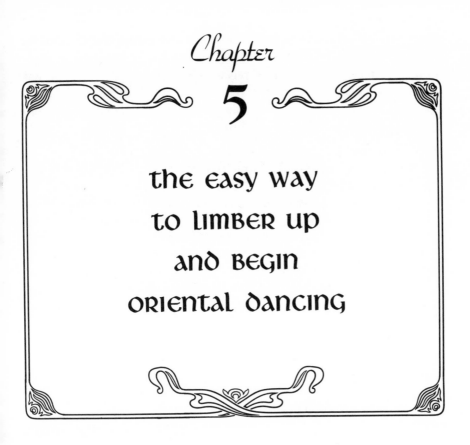

Chapter

5

the easy way
to LimBER up
and BeGin
ORiental dancing

The body is a glorious temple that must be shined, polished, nourished properly, and be looked upon with awe and respect. Otherwise the human body will start to tarnish and rot away like so many present-day structures that builders choose to build with inferior materials. Buildings are built of concrete, bricks, wood, and other materials. The ones that stay with us, barring acts of God, are the ones that are built upon solid ground with solid materials. Likewise, the body should be built solidly with proper nutrition, exercise, and other healthy habits.

Proper exercise and sensible eating patterns are the raw materials for building a firm, exciting body; otherwise, it too will fade away into antiquity. In keeping with this idea we start off on our road to a healthier, happier body with what I like to call "body stretches."

You "stretch" your mind through various learning processes. If you fill your mind with undesirable information, chances are it will slowly deteriorate. By the same token, if you leave your body in a dormant, unfed state, never exercising a muscle except when you get up from the chair in front of the television set to go to bed in the bedroom, your body is sure to follow the same deteriorating process that an unexercised mind goes through.

YOUR FLEXIBLE BODY

Your body was made to move. If it weren't you would be as immovable as a statue, without any joints at all. If your joints could only move stiffly, you would move something like the Tin Man in the "Wizard of Oz" or like some other weird-looking machine-person. Instead, you have wonderfully flexible joints, and I think that you owe it to yourself to keep these joints in tip-top condition. After all, life is motion, and the better shape your joints are in, the better you'll be able to move and enjoy life.

Before you get to the body-building form of controlled, systematic Oriental dance exercises, it is necessary for you to limber up and make your body more flexible so that you will build up an ease with which you can bend your body more effortlessly without aches or pains or other damaging problems when you do your Oriental dance exercises.

HOW YOGA CAN HELP

You may limber up with the stretching exercises I suggested in Chapter 1, or you may prefer to try some yoga movements. Lately I have been "turned on" to Hatha Yoga and have been doing the exercises (asanas) to limber up my body. Hatha Yoga was something I wanted to do for a very long time, but I never made the time for it. You know how you can find every conceivable excuse to prevent you from doing certain things. A friend once told me that anyone can find time to do things if that person wants to do them. Well, finally, one day a girlfriend of mine told me about a yoga class that she had found. She told me what a serene feeling she had gotten from going there and how it made her relax completely. This sounded like Nirvana to me, so I figured that I would join her there and check it out myself. Well, all I can say is that I have missed only one week since then. My Hatha Yoga class is written into my calendar as if it were a permanent part of me, and indeed I do feel that it is a part of my being. It's hard to explain the calmness that the yoga exercises (asanas or postures) bring to your body and your mind. It just happens—your body and mind take on a beautiful spiritual condition.

The asanas are coordinated with your breathing and are never strained. You seem to bring new life to your body in the form of a peace that you never knew before. You become aware of your breathing, that very life force without which you would be nothing. The breathing exercises help rid your body of all the impurities that you can't help but inhale from the air you breathe, especially if you live in a large metropolitan area.

USING YOGA FOR WARMING UP

If you wish, you can use some yoga asanas as your warm-up exercises. Remember that you should never push yourself too far. You may feel some discomfort doing something for the first time, but that's something that will go away after you become more proficient at it. However, if you feel any pain please do not continue the asana. You keep the poses at a point where you feel comfortable with them. Overdoing them and straining your body when it is not ready will only lead to trouble. In yoga you never strain your body, and all your asanas are performed in a flowing motion so as not to damage your body.

The one exercise that I would like to include here for your benefit is the yoga Salutation to the Sun. It is an almost complete exercise (asana) in that every part of the body gets "oiled" and stretched. It is called Sun Salutation because after you're through you can feel the warmth of the sun in your entire body. It is therefore a great warm-up exercise for you to do before you get into the Oriental dance exercises. Yoga will bring your body, mind, and spirit into one and will start energy flowing to all parts of the body.

In yoga, breathing is an integral part, as I said before, so I have included breathing instructions where necessary so that you can perform this asana as correctly as possible. All movements should be done slowly and smoothly. Whenever you achieve a new position, hold it for a second before proceeding. Later on I will give you some other limbering up exercises.

These are just a few of the things that I have learned about Hatha Yoga. If you take up yoga you will enjoy it too. I love doing my asanas with my yogi because his quiet voice guiding me through the asanas adds a new dimension to them for me.

Sun Salutation

- Assume a standing position.
- Feet together, bend knees slightly, hands at sides, legs straight.
- Bend elbows and place hands together at chest level in a praying position—palms of hands together, fingers pointing towards ceiling.
- Slowly raise both hands straight up over your head, palms facing forward.
- Bend head backwards as far as you can comfortably and look up at hands, *inhale*.
- Slowly bend over forwards and try to touch the floor with your hands, *exhale*.
- Place palms of hands on floor if you can.
- Bend knees and stoop down, placing right leg straight out, knee on floor, behind you; other leg remains bent.
- Bend head backwards and *inhale*.
- Stretch left leg back and stretch body out straight, arms are straight, feet together, hold.
- Curl toes under, drop knees, then chest, to floor, fanny stays up, *exhale*.
- Lay flat on floor, hold head back, *inhale*.
- Bring feet up and leave hands on floor, fanny up in the air as if someone were pulling you up by it, *exhale*.
- Stretch left foot back and place knee on floor.
- Bend right knee and hold it right under your chest, hands still on floor.
- Bend head backwards, *inhale*.
- Bring left knee up to right knee.
- Push yourself up, keeping head near to knee, *exhale*.
- Slowly rise to a standing position, hands straight up over head.
- Bend head and hands backwards, *inhale*.
- Return hands to praying position, head straight, *exhale*.
- Repeat two times (increase gradually to six times when comfortable).

Every time you move, muscles in your body are contracting. These are groups of thin little fibers that respond to stimulation by the method of contracting and then springing back to their original state.

Think of a muscle as an elastic band. When you squeeze, stretch, or twist it, it returns to its original shape. Your muscles will become more elastic after a few stretches. This is why it is necessary for you to stretch them gently before you go into any rigorous exercise. This will give your muscles good muscle tone, which gives them a firm quality. Technically, you do not stretch your muscles when you exercise; that is why I call this next set of exercises body stretches instead of muscle stretches. I love the idea of stretching my body because it gives me the feeling that I am really limbering up and "oiling" my joints, and you know how creaky they can get when you don't use them.

Your skeletal muscles supply mobility for the body, so you have to keep them in tone. To do this you have to stretch the ligaments to make your joints more limber. Would you believe that you have, considering that you have a mature body, more than 600 muscles in your body? If you don't use your muscles they will shrink and waste away—all 600 of them.

DOING REGULAR BODY STRETCHES

These body stretches can be done every other day in their entirety if you are trying to maintain your weight. If you are trying to lose weight, do all the body stretches or about 20 minutes of the other miscellaneous exercises in this chapter at night before you go to bed, or some other time in the evening. You will therefore be exercising in the mornings with your Oriental dance exercises and at night with the complete set of body stretches. Everyone should do about 10 minutes of these body stretches before they start their Oriental dance exercises. This way your body will be stretched and ready for your concentrated exercises. Remember that you have the alternative of doing the Hatha Yoga asanas to limber up. I would like you to alternate the Sun Salutation with the body stretches before you do your Oriental dance exercises. One of the goals should be to achieve good muscle tone. In order to do this it will be necessary for you to exercise all your muscles. Muscle tone is the state of firmness of a muscle. Don't be afraid if a little soreness occurs when you do your exercises. This happens when the least-trained muscle fibers in your body are irritated or when the muscles that you have been using during your exercises are irritated for one reason or another. With constant exercise this will disappear.

If you don't use your muscles, they will atrophy. It is therefore important for you to use your muscles if you want them to develop well. If you get muscle cramps because of misuse or whatever, just firmly knead the affected area. They will go away after awhile.

The strength of your muscles can be built up and developed by exercising them against some sort of resistance. I like to exercise using water as the resistance because it is fun; however, weights or springs can be used. Don't forget that each person develops at his or her own pace, so don't be discouraged if you don't achieve all your goals overnight. You will achieve them at your own pace.

It is most important that you keep up your exercises and do not neglect them, because when you stop exercising, your appetite remains the same, and since you are expending less energy, you will gain weight.

Pearl L. was an Oriental dance student of mine. She started taking my classes to try to lose 25 pounds. I felt it was my duty to inform her that those 25 pounds would be with her forever if she thought that an appearance once a week in my class was the magic wand that would make them disappear. I immediately introduced her to my program of systematic weight loss and exercise. After 5 weeks she lost all her unwanted pounds. Three years later she's still maintaining her desired weight.

WHEN YOUR MOVEMENTS BECOME REFLEXES

Remember that practice becomes perfect. If you practice conscientiously you will improve your dexterity, and before long your exercises will become second nature to you. These movements can become almost as simple, routine, and as quick as a reflex action. Speaking of reflexes, this subject reminds me of one day when I visited the doctor's office for a regular checkup. He was checking my reflexes by tapping my knee with that little instrument that looks like a hammer. Nothing happened folks. My foot just stayed there and did not move at all. No reaction, no reflexes. "What did that mean?" I thought to myself. Finally, I said to the doctor, "Why don't you put on some Middle Eastern music, I'll show you reflexes." I had finally gotten my doctor to crack a smile. I guess that each person reacts to different stimuli. Maybe I had this reaction because I am so involved with Oriental dancing that I thought that was the answer. It turned out okay though, because he eventually found the secret spot—and up went the foot. It was a relief to find out that I do have reflexes after all! Prior to this I thought that the only place that the doctor could tap was the knee, but there are other places folks! You really do learn something new every day.

This was a funny situation, but it also leads to another point that I want to make about my exercises. It has been proven that music acts as a reinforcing stimulus which will make you exercise more energetically, and even though you are expending more energy, the exercise will become easier to you. That is why I would recommend that you always exercise to music.

You get the energy that you need for muscular work from the food you eat. It is said that you get energy from carbohydrates, fats, and proteins. So you see that it is important to have a well-balanced eating pattern so that you will have the energy to do your exercises.

This next paragraph bears repeating. You should never strain yourself doing any sort of exercise. Only you can tell just how far you can push your body. Only you can tell the difference between being uncomfortable and suffering outright pain. If you experience the latter, please do not pursue the exercises. The idea is gradually to work your body into them, not to shock your body.

Most women think of their breasts as muscles; however, your breasts are glands, not muscles. Once these glands become flabby, only a plastic surgeon can correct the condition. However, you can at that point in time work on strengthening your pectoral (chest) muscles to obtain a firmer look. The cup size of your breast will not increase, but the pectoral muscles under the breast can be developed and your overall chest area can be increased.

The greatest and easiest way to have your breasts appear larger is to maintain good posture. If you slouch, your breasts will get lost in your caved-in upper torso. Straighten out those shoulders, and you will add miraculous, illusionary inches to your bustline. Try this and you will be truly amazed at the difference a simple thing like correct posture can make to your bustline.

To help your pectoral muscles get firm and to tone up the chest area, do the following exercises whenever you get a chance—when you go to the bathroom, when you shower, while you watch TV, or whenever.

Firmness Exercise#1

- Assume a correct posture (standing erect, shoulders back, chin up, feet slightly apart).
- Raise your hands in front of you to shoulder level.
- Bring palms together in a praying position, elbows at shoulder level, fingertips straight up towards the ceiling.

- Push against palms and hold for a count of 5, then relax.
- Repeat 15 times.

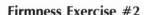

Firmness Exercise #2

- Assume a seated position.
- Head and back straight.
- Hands at sides.
- Place your hands behind your back and grasp your fingers in an interlocking position.
- Let hands touch your fanny.
- Slowly raise arms behind you as high as you can.
- Hold for count of 5.
- Slowly lower your arms.
- Repeat slowly 5 times (increase to 10 times when comfortable).

Firmness Exercise # 3

- Lie flat on the floor, face down, hands straight out at sides perpendicular to your body.
- Push up your whole body until only your hands and toes are touching the floor.
- Hold for a count of 5.
- Return to lying position and relax.
- Repeat pushups slowly about 5 times, more when you feel comfortable.

Exercise #3 will take a little more energy and stamina, so do not overdo it and strain yourself. If you can manage only one pushup the first day, fine. There is always tomorrow to increase them.

IMPROVING THE BUSTLINE

One of the Oriental dancer's assets is a firm bustline and one that is fairly visible. You too can work on developing and toning this part of your body. An Oriental dancer's costume for her cabaret performance is rather revealing. One of the parts of the body that seems to catch people's attention the most is the bustline. In my opinion it is always nice to see a great bustline. Some dancers wear push-up bras to emphasize their bustline a little more. In our society, in spite of the women's liberation movement, men, and indeed women too, still admire a nice full bustline. This is a great asset to an Oriental dancer; however, it is definitely not a prerequisite as some people think. So many women come up to me and make some kind of remark to the effect that they could never be an Oriental dancer because their busts are too small. Wrong. Some of the finest dancers I know have rather modest bustlines. With this thought in mind, let us talk a little bit more about busts for a minute. Don't expect miracles from the firmness exercises. If you develop the proper attitude in terms of your posture and projection of yourself, it will not only show in your bustline but it will show all over your body. Over a period of six months you should see some visible changes in the appearance of your bustline if you exercise faithfully.

STRANGE EXPERIENCES

At this point I have to tell you some of the stories that happened to me because of my bustline. Fortunately, or should I say unfortunately for me, I have a pretty full bustline. Needless to say I have had to endure more than my share of "bust jokes." Anyway, I have tried to be good-natured about them and not let the jokes bother me. I just take them in stride.

One of my first strange experiences as an Oriental dancer had to do with a curious man showing up in my dressing room after my show to see if my bust was "real." Of course he scared me half to death, but I sized him up pretty quickly and I realized he wasn't crazy or anything like that; he was genuinely curious. His curiosity was so genuine it was a little sad. I did my best to satisfy his curiosity without stripping, but the whole situation was really weird. How would you like to walk into your dressing room and be confronted with a guy standing there saying, "Are they real, are they, I gotta find out, are they real?" At first I couldn't figure out whether he was talking about my hair, my eyelashes, or what. It didn't take me too long to find out just what he was talking about. It was a very funny, and at the same time sort of a sad evening for me, but it turned out okay, thank goodness. This incident made me check that my dressing room doors all had locks on them from then on.

This brings to mind another story which is hard to categorize as to whether it is funny or pathetic. I always try to look on the humorous side of things because it seems that it helps me through life. During my show one night I had done a back bend beside this guy in the audience, and there were my breasts looking him straight in the eye, or was it vice versa? With that he said, "Don't come any closer or I'll bite them." Well, he looked well fed to me, and besides, guys were always threatening me with things like that and none ever carried out the threat. This is just their way of showing how aggressive and "manly" (?) they are. Well, this one carried out his threat! Of course panic set in. I thought for sure I would get cancer of the breast, or rabies at the very least. I laughed (while crying and shrieking inside) and finished my show. The show must go on! After the show there was a knock on the door while I was calling my mother, doctor, veterinarian, the Mayo Clinic, and you name it. Should I call my gynecologist, my internist, my orthopedic surgeon—help, who takes care of breasts? I opened the door and there was the same guy, sober as a judge, and out came an apology the length of my arm. With that he handed me a hundred dollar bill. After I had said, "Oh, think nothing of it, it was just an accident," I said with as straight a face as I could muster, "Would you like to bite the other one?" We started to laugh and that was that. No, he didn't get a second nibble, but he had sobered up a lot.

MY BIGGEST TRAUMA

Of course the biggest trauma in an Oriental dancer's life is the fear of having a bra strap snap. This has happened to me only twice in my many years of dancing. Fortunately for me, both times I was able to fix it before the whole audience was aware of what was happening. Even the musicians didn't get wind of it because I was working in places where I had worked for a long time and the musicians played my show sort of automatically. A lot of musicians have the knack of never noticing that you are on the stage if you have been working with them for any length of time. Many an Oriental dancer will vouch for that. I have often been tempted just to lie there on the stage, stiff as a doornail, and see whether they would continue playing my music without noticing that I was prostrate. Anyway, back to our exercises.

Since each of you is different, it is important for you to approach any exercise program with caution. I don't want you to strain yourself doing any exercises, because the idea is to help you not to injure you or cause you discomfort. So therefore, when you perform your exercises, if you experience any stress, such as tension, slight trembling or shortness of breath, or any unusual symptoms, don't push yourself. Remember that Rome wasn't built in a day.

BEFORE YOU EXERCISE

Remember that before you start any exercise routine, even the simple body stretches, you should have a checkup by a qualified doctor so that he can tell you whether you are in the best physical condition to reap the exercise benefit. We don't want any ruptured parts of your body lying on the floor next to you after you have done fifteen minutes of exercises. Each body responds differently to various stimuli, so who is better to advise you than your personal physician who knows your body inside out? If you are getting on in years it wouldn't hurt to take a stress test. This just checks how your heart reacts to physical exercise. It shows how much effort you should put forth during your exercises. It can also bring to light any hidden disease. You don't want to put undue strain on yourself.

Exercise stimulates digestion, but you should not eat for at least one hour before you start any exercises, be they yoga or other limbering up exercises, or Oriental dance exercises. I follow this rule and so do the majority of dancers I know. Most dancers also do not eat at least one hour before an actual performance. I know a few dancers who will eat a heavy meal and then go right on the stage and perform for a strenuous 20 minutes and more. This is very damaging for your digestion and for your health. You could experience muscle cramps and a great deal of pain if you exercise on a full stomach. Just try to imagine your food being shaken and rolled like wet clothes tumbling in a dryer.

STARTING GRADUALLY

Here's another word of caution: Do not overdo the exercises. You start off gradually by exercising for only a few minutes each day at a specific time set aside by yourself. If you make a habit of this, the exercises will come much easier and you can build up to a more intensive program as time goes by. I find that mornings are a good time to exercise. After you have stumbled out of bed it is a great eye opener, and before you know it you'll be rolling out of bed doing your exercises without a second thought. Of course, if you are on a reducing eating pattern you will have to exercise in the mornings as well as in the evenings before you go to bed. You should set aside times in the day when you can best fit this into your schedule without too much rescheduling of your life. If you have a family, think of their needs and schedule your exercise time when they least need you because you don't want to be interrupted while doing your exercises. The ideal thing to do would be to let them do the exercises with you.

It is important that you bring the proper attitude with you to your exercise time. Leave all your cares aside and come to your exercises with a relaxed feeling. Open your mind to a spiritual and physical aura of well-being. You will be surprised how this attitude can help you not only with your exercises but also in giving you a new outlook on life. You should become a more serene person, and in this age of stressful situations, pressures, and deadlines to meet, it is imperative that you relax more and take good care of yourself. Remember, nobody else is going to do it for you.

A POSITIVE ATTITUDE

A positive attitude can be developed with some perseverance on your part. First of all, you must keep telling yourself over and over that you will succeed in your goals. I have found that my positive attitude towards life has moved mountains for me. For example, when I had the idea for this book I tried to share it with a few of my friends. Most of them said, "Great, go ahead and write it." A few were very discouraging to say the least. They couldn't believe that I would actually write a book. Had I listened to them and their negativism, I wouldn't have been able to express myself and you wouldn't have had a chance to buy this book and benefit from it. I simply ignored the negative thinking and went straight ahead with my project. I set a goal for myself and stuck to it and succeeded. You can do it too. You must do it.

This positive attitude can get you through anything in life—through your marriage, your job, your everyday life, and through your exercises. Just try giving yourself a pep talk if you find yourself slipping into negativism. Think positively and everything will be positive. Most important of all, shed your negative thinking friends. If you can't do that totally, be sure not to let their negative thinking stop you from doing anything you want to do in this world. Maybe you will make a few mistakes, but on the whole you will achieve your goals. Again, think positively—you learn by your mistakes. That's what makes achievement so rewarding. Everybody makes mistakes, even the very rich and beautiful. The trick is to try to minimize them. Put your mind to it and do it. Bring a positive attitude to your exercises and you will succeed. Just keep repeating, "I can do it. I will do it." You will do it. You will lose the weight you want to lose.

You don't need too much courage to get started. Just follow the simple steps listed below and don't stop to contemplate, rehash, and talk yourself out of doing your exercises. Just do them.

First, you should slip into something comfortable. Leotards and tights, body suits, bathing suits, or if you're a completely free person, just bring your body minus the trimmings.

Second, get your records and record player ready. I have found a better way of doing this than fooling around with records and record players. Get your tape recorder and tape all the songs onto a cassette, slow tunes on one side and fast tunes on the other side. This saves time because you do not have to jump from record to record looking for specific tempos. This will come in handy, especially for the Oriental dance exercises. For the body stretches you'll use the slow Middle Eastern tunes or any other type of slow, relaxing music.

Third, you must clear your mind of all your problems. You must bring a trouble-free mind to your exercise period.

Fourth, take a few deep breaths, inhale and exhale about ten times. (See Breathing Exercise below.) Let your hands hang loose, shake them vigorously, relax your entire body, then relax your feet and shake them, one foot at a time, of course. If you can do two feet at a time, throw away this book because you're a better person than I and I should be taking lessons from you!

Fifth, maintaining correct posture during all your exercises is most important. This was explained fully in Chapter 1.

Breathing Exercise

- Assume correct posture.
- Inhale a deep breath.
- Pull in abdomen and lift rib cage high and hold breath for a count of 5.
- Lower rib cage and exhale very slowly.
- Repeat 10 times.

BODY STRETCHING EXERCISES

The body stretches that follow should be done for approximately 20 minutes if you are on a weight-reducing program, and they can form a whole exercise routine of their own. If you have a great deal of weight to lose, these body stretches can serve as a supplemental exercise routine. If you are on a maintaining routine, do them for about 10 minutes. Do them in the order in which they are listed here. Remember, the objective is to stretch the various parts of your body and to limber them up. When you finish these stretches, your body will be tingling with excitement and it will be ready for just about anything, and most of all, for your Oriental dance exercises.

When you do these body stretches before your Oriental dance exercises, do each one only once to limber up your body. Remember, the body stretches should be done very slowly in order to reap the most benefits from them.

Body stretches are very good to relieve the aches and pains that your body sometimes experiences. They also loosen up your joints and muscles and stimulate your circulation. Whenever you get a moment, you can do a few of them to sort of "wake you up." They increase your energy and your endurance and provide an overall beautiful toning effect to your body.

Scalp Stretch

- Assume any relaxed seated position.
- Grab a firm hold of large clumps of hair at the roots, first to the front, then to the back of the head.
- Move scalp gently back and forth.
- Repeat about 10 times.

Neck Stretch (backwards)

- Assume correct posture.
- Hold head erect, hands at sides.
- Slowly stretch head and neck backwards as far as possible.
- Hold for count of 10.
- Increase to count of 15 after a few days.
- Repeat a few times.

Neck Stretch (frontal)

- Assume correct posture.
- Hold head erect.
- Bend forward until chin touches chest.
- Hold for count of 10.
- Increase to count of 15 after a few days.
- Repeat a few times.

Neck Stretch (sidewards)

- Assume correct posture.
- Hold head erect.
- Bend head over to the left until cheek almost touches shoulder.
- Hold for count of 10.
- Increase to count of 15 after a few days.
- Repeat same exercise on the right side.
- Repeat a few times.

Shoulder Stretch

- Assume correct posture.
- Place hands on shoulders.
- Stretch elbows back until shoulder blades almost touch.
- Hold for count of 10.
- Increase to count of 15 after a few days.
- Repeat a few times.

Elbow, Shoulder, Spine Stretch (backwards)

- Assume correct posture.
- Arms at sides.
- Slowly raise arms, palms facing outward, to shoulder level.
- Lower arms and swing them to the back.
- Interlock fingers.
- Slowly bend head backwards, chest follows.
- Slowly bend forward to upright position.
- Bring arms up.

- Hold for count of 10.
- Increase to a count of 15 after a few days.
- Repeat a few times.

Spine Stretch (forwards)

- Assume correct posture.
- Arms at sides.
- Slowly lower head until chin touches neck.
- Bring hands forward.
- Keep lowering head.
- Shoulders come forward, back bends slowly.
- Continue to bend back until head just hangs there.
- Hang loose and relax for count of 10.
- Increase to count of 15 after a few days.
- Slowly straighten up to starting position.
- Repeat a few times.

Back and Spine Stretch (a)

- Sit on floor, legs together and outstretched.
- Rest hands on thighs.
- Slowly raise arms to shoulder level.
- Bring arms over head.
- Then bend forward.
- Lower arms and hold knees tightly.
- Pull trunk down as far as possible.
- Elbows bend out.
- Hold for count of 10.
- Increase to count of 15 after a few days.
- Repeat a few times.

Back and Spine Stretch (b)

- Lie on floor, face down.
- Hands at sides, chin on the floor.
- Slowly place hands under shoulders.
- Raise head slowly.
- Push hands on floor, then elbows bend slowly, thus raising trunk.
- Spine should be curved.

- Tilt head back.
- Hold for count of 10.
- Increase to a count of 15 after a few days.
- Repeat a few times.

Waist Stretch

- Assume correct posture.
- Feet about one foot apart.
- Raise arms to sides, shoulder level, palms facing down.
- Swing right arm down slowly over the left side as far as possible.
- Hold left knee with left hand.
- Knees are straight.
- Hold for a count of 10.
- Increase to count of 15 after a few days.
- Slowly straighten to starting position.
- Repeat on the other side.
- Hold for a count of 10.
- Increase to a count of 15 after a few days.
- Repeat a few times.

Knee and Thigh Stretch

- Assume seated position on floor.
- Feet straight out in front.
- Bend knees and bring feet up to your buttocks.
- Grasp front of legs with hands and press thighs to your chest.
- Lower legs as close to floor as possible (about 1" off floor).
- Hold back straight up.
- Hold for a count of 10.
- Increase to a count of 15 after a few days.
- Repeat a few times.

Leg Stretch

- Assume correct posture.
- Lie on floor on right side.
- Right hand at side, left hand resting on left leg.
- Lift left leg slowly as far as possible.
- Point toes.

- Hold for count of 10.
- Slowly lower leg.
- Repeat on the left side, raising right leg slowly.
- Hold for a count of 10.
- Increase to count of 15 after a few days.
- Repeat a few times.

Hand Stretch

- Assume correct posture.
- Hands to sides.
- Slowly raise arms to shoulder level, straight out in front.
- Palms open face down, spread fingers and stretch them out, opened as far as possible, hold.
- Slowly close fingers until tightly closed.
- Hold for a count of 10.
- Repeat three times.
- Increase to count of 15 after a few days.

Finger Stretch

- Assume correct posture.
- Hands at sides.
- Bend arms at elbows.
- Take the right hand and pull each finger of the left hand (you'll sometimes hear a cracking sound).
- Do the same thing with the left hand.
- Repeat for about one minute.

HOW ORIENTAL DANCERS EXERCISE

Needless to say, not all Oriental dancers do these body stretches before they exercise; however, they are some of the commonly used limbering up exercises.

It was Machiavelli who said that there is no one way of realizing absolute truth. Taking this a little further, I would like to say that there is no one form of exercise that is the absolute exercise. For this reason I have questioned several dancers on what form their physical fitness routines took. Not surprisingly they came up with a number of various answers.

Oriental dancers, like any other group of people or dance professionals, have their own individual ways of keeping in shape. Some of my friends work out at gyms on a regular basis, some dancers do karate, and some dancers do a lot of walking, swimming, jogging, bicycling, calisthenics, or even another dance form like ballet or jazz dancing. Actually, no matter what form your exercise takes, the important thing is that you do it on a regular basis and let it become a regular part of your life style. If you exercise your body in a sporadic manner, your body is going to react to this in a negative way. If you do your exercises on an ongoing basis, your body is going to respond accordingly and you will have a "machine" that will not break down and will not be in need of constant "repair."

One exercise I haven't tried yet is jogging. It is an excellent form of exercise. Many of my Oriental dance friends practice this form of exercise. The people who are really into it will jog anywhere.

When you jog you metabolize fat, and this is replaced by muscle tissue. It is good for the lungs and heart. First you should start with short runs and build up your tolerance slowly. Stay away from traffic fumes which are dangerous to your lungs.

Women will be glad to hear that this exercise, as well as other forms of exercise, helps to relax the uterine muscles, which helps to avoid painful days during the menstrual period.

You often hear people say, "Oh, I exercise but it doesn't help." Well, I can bet you that those people have not exercised religiously for any period of time. I know this as a fact because at times I have been guilty of that very same irresponsibility. You must exercise regularly to reap the benefits.

Good posture and a keen sense of balance are most important to dancers. It's funny but I am like a real "klutz" (clumsy) when I am offstage. On stage, my two left feet seem to straighten out and glide around the stage as if they were built to do only that. All of a sudden I become Miss Graceful.

Many dancers do a balancing act as part of their dance routine. I saw a Moroccan male dancer do a fantastic balancing act when I was visiting Tangiers. Many Middle Eastern dancers, especially the Moroccan dancers, balance filled glasses on their heads, but this was the first time I saw someone balance a filled goblet and a dozen glasses filled with water on a well-arranged tray. He did this with such precision, it was amazing. He twirled around like a whirlwind. He even did this balancing act while twisting his body around on the floor, without spilling so much as a drop of the liquid. He also did some other very interesting balancing feats that were mind-boggling. Picture, if you can, this one. He placed a full glass of water in each hand, and, with arms outstretched, proceeded to spin like a top. The glasses were just being held there with a prayer because these glasses were perpendicular to the palms of his hands. I still don't know how he did this.

Posture

- Stand erect with a fairly heavy book on your head.
- Hands out at sides, perpendicular to your body.
- Eyes straight forward and focus on something at eye level to keep your balance.
- Walk around the room, keeping your head straight for about one-and-a-half minutes (count to 100).

Here are some of the other exercises that my dancer friends do to keep in shape for their Oriental dancing. These are exercises that they do in addition to their Oriental dance routines. These can help put the spice of variety into your life.

Dumbbells Exercise # 1

You can pick up a fairly light pair for these exercises in any sporting goods store. Exercises are sometimes much more beneficial when you exercise against some form of resistance such as using weights. Many exercises can be done while holding the dumbbells. Here are just a few simple ones for you. Dancers who do this do it to build tone rather than strength. Men who lift weights do it to build strength.

- Lie flat on your back on the floor.
- Feet straight out.
- Arms extended straight to each side, perpendicular to body with dumbbells in hands.

- Raise dumbbells slowly until your hands are together above you.
- Push hands together and hold for count of 2.
- Slowly lower hands and return them to the floor.
- Repeat 5 times (increase to 10 times when comfortable).

Dumbbells Exercise # 2

- Stand erect with hands at sides, holding dumbbells.
- Slowly bring hands up to the shoulders and bend elbows.
- Hold for a count of 2.
- Then straighten arms and hold dumbbells overhead.
- Hold for count of 2.
- Lower hands to shoulders.
- Hold for count of 2.
- Then lower arms to the sides.
- Repeat 5 times (increase to 10 when comfortable).

Dumbbells Exercise # 3

- Stand erect with hands at sides holding dumbbells.
- Slowly bring arms up to shoulder level and continue in a circle until arms are above your head.
- Hold for count of 2.
- Slowly lower arms to starting position.
- Repeat 5 times (increase to 10 when comfortable).

Backward Knee Bends

- Assume a kneeling position on all fours.
- Gradually straighten the left leg out in back.
- Bend knees and grab hold of the ankles with the left hand and pull leg towards your head as far as possible.
- Hold for count of 2.
- Return leg to the floor, kneeling position.
- Repeat the same thing with your right foot and right hand.
- Return leg to floor.

- Repeat 5 times on each side (increase to 10 times when comfortable).
- Be careful with this exercise, it's a little tricky.

Leg Raises

- Stand straight, slowly bend over and hold on to the back of a tall chair, bureau, or exercise bar.
- Back should be parallel to the floor.
- Feet together.
- Slowly raise the right leg backwards as far as it will go.
- Hold for a count of 2.
- Return to floor.
- Repeat with left leg.
- Hold for count of 2.
- Slowly alternate legs about 5 times (increase to 10 times when comfortable).

This exercise can also be done raising legs out to the sides instead of straight back.

Hand Exercise, Curling Fingers

- Sit on a chair.
- Extend hands out in front of you, fingers stretched out, palms facing downwards.
- Close fingers and make a tight fist.
- Hold for count of 2.
- Relax and repeat 10 times.

This can also be done with palms facing upwards.

Circular Arm Rotation

- Assume standing position.
- Raise hands to sides, extended perpendicular to the body.
- Keeping elbows straight, rotate arms in small circular motions clockwise.
- Repeat 10 times.

- Then rotate arms counterclockwise.
- Repeat 10 times.

This is a good exercise for the shoulders and the back.

Foot Exercise, Pointing Toes

- Sit on a chair and extend feet out in front of you parallel to the floor, toes pointing straight up.
- Place hands at sides, holding chair seat.
- Point toes backwards toward your body.
- Hold for count of 2.
- Then point toes down toward the ground.
- Hold for count of 2.
- Repeat 10 times.

You can also do this by alternating feet.

Alternate Leg Raises

- Sit on a chair and extend feet out in front of you parallel to the floor.
- Point toes.
- Hands at sides holding chair seat.
- Raise right leg up in the air as far as you can comfortably go.
- Lower to original position.
- Raise left leg up in the air as far as you can comfortably go.
- Alternate feet slowly in a scissor-like motion.
- Do this for about 1 minute.

Touching Toes (Standing)

- Stand erect, hands at sides.
- Slowly bend over and touch your toes.
- Legs should be bent slightly.
- Stay there for count of 5.
- Slowly return to standing position.
- Repeat slowly 5 times (increase to 10 when comfortable).

Touching Toes (Seated)

- Assume a seated position on the floor.
- Legs together, straight out in front of you.
- Hands resting on knees.
- Slowly bend forward and try to touch your toes.
- Keep your head bent down.
- Go as far as you can without straining yourself.
- Repeat 5 times (increase to 10 when comfortable).

This is definitely one of those exercises in which you will see some progress as you get better at it.

Touching Shins in Mid Air

- Lie flat on your back.
- Feet together and straight out in front.
- Arms straight out over your head.
- Slowly raise feet and arms off the floor until they are straight up, perpendicular to floor.
- Try to touch your legs, but do not strain yourself.
- Slowly return hands and feet to floor.
- Repeat 5 times (increase to 10 when comfortable).

Swimming Exercise # 1—The Australian Crawl

Note: Swimming is one of the best forms of exercise and one that is also a lot of fun. Many people can't get to a beach area or a swimming pool too easily, so I thought that I would simulate some of the basic strokes used in swimming so that you can do them in the privacy of your own home. If you have access to a body of water, by all means try to swim every day.

- Get a large sturdy hassock and place it in an unencumbered area so that you will have room to stretch.
- Lie flat on your stomach, making sure to balance yourself.
- Body straight and hands at sides.
- Slowly bend right elbow and bring your hand along your side.

- Slowly bring hand around in a circular motion and stretch it straight ahead.
- Slowly return arm to starting position.
- Do the same thing with your left hand.
- Then alternate hands in an Australian crawl motion.
- When your left hand is back, your right hand should be forward in an alternating motion.
- When your left hand is stretched forward, turn your head to the right side.
- When your right hand is stretched forward, turn your head to the left side.
- Repeat 5 times (increase to 10 when comfortable).

Swimming Exercise # 2—Breast Stroke

- Get a large sturdy hassock and place it in an unencumbered area so that you will have room to stretch.
- Lie flat on your stomach, making sure to balance yourself.
- Body straight and hands at sides.
- Head and feet straight out.
- Slowly bring both hands along your sides until they reach your chest.
- Push hands straight out in front of you.
- Make a semi-circle with both hands until hands are perpendicular to your body.
- Bend elbows and return hands to chest.
- Repeat breast stroke 5 times (increase to 10 when comfortable).

Swimming Exercise # 3—Back Stroke, Seated

- Sit on a sturdy hassock.
- Hands at your sides.
- Hold feet straight out and flap them up and down.
- Slowly raise right hand up in front of you until it is shoulder level.
- Bring it straight up in a semi-circular motion until the inside of your elbow is by your ear.
- Continue this circular motion backwards until your hand is back at your side.

- Do the same with the left hand.
- Alternate hands in a windmill motion.
- Repeat 5 times (increase to 10 when comfortable).

For variety you could do it with both hands together. This exercise could also be done in a standing position.

A BRIEF HISTORY OF ORIENTAL DANCING

Before I go any further, I think that it is most important that you become familiar with a little history of the Oriental dance. This is important so that you are not doing these exercises in a vacuum. When you do yoga you become familiar with the philosophy behind it so that you can truly appreciate it. The same thing goes for any other dance form or discipline. Then you can go full speed ahead and immerse yourself to your full potential and understanding of the dance.

Through the research that I have done, I have come to the conclusion that the Oriental dance was done in pre-Biblical days and perhaps goes back to the beginning of time. Did Eve do an Oriental dance for Adam?

Archaeological excavations have given us some insight into the dance. The paintings in the ancient Egyptian tombs and temples often reveal a dancer in some pose related to the Oriental dance. The arm movements that we use today are definitely related to the ancient Egyptian arm positions. Recently, I visited the Palazzo Carignano in Turin, Italy, to see the Egyptian collection and was none too surprised to see these pictures of dancers firsthand. The Kunsthistorisches Museum in Vienna, Austria, also has an important Egyptian collection. Mention should also be made of the National Museum in Naples, Italy. A museum closer to home which has a large Egyptian collection would be the Metropolitan Museum of Art in New York City, where you can browse through its Egyptian collection with fascination.

In Biblical times, Salome danced for Herod and his birthday guests. The Bible tells us that, " . . . the daughter of Herodias danced before them and pleased Herod." That's where the dance of the seven veils originated in case you're wondering.

Through the centuries, many have conjured up their own versions of Salome's famous dance (even actress Rita Hayworth had her turn at it) until today most anyone would say that her movements resembled those of the Oriental dance movements. The dance probably originated in Persia, the birthplace of the oud, that delightful instrument that gives so much life to the Oriental dance. Then the Turks got into the act and spread it throughout Egypt, which they ruled for hundreds of years. There is no doubt in my mind as to the great influence that the ancient Egyptian dances have on the Oriental dance today. Many dancers and interested parties are doing a great deal of research on the Oriental dance, and more and more historical facts are coming to the fore lately. However, we still have a long way to go.

DANCING IN RELIGION

The dance has been part of the ritual of various religions—dances have been done to praise the gods and to placate them. For the most part these dances comprised a swaying of the body in all directions and the use of the hands to extend the motion. Dancers have provided entertainment in the palaces and courts of the Pharaohs and the kings and queens of the world from ancient times.

The Middle Eastern culture is one that hangs onto its traditions, which go unchanged for centuries, so it's not too farfetched a notion to presume that the Oriental dance that has come from the Middle East is not too dissimilar from dances done there thousands of years ago.

The dance was banned in the 1800's in Egypt. When it started to flourish again, the dancers had to cover their bodies from head to toe. As it gained a little more "respectability," the dancers got daring and began to show a little more. They would cover their midriff with fine netting, but you could see through this fabric. It's interesting how "modesty" takes many different forms depending upon which area you are in. In certain cultures it's acceptable for you to have your breasts naked, in others that's a definite "no-no." In Egypt, the Pharaonic dancing girls wore a lot less than other dancers. Maybe the Pharaohs were wise men after all!

When Gamal Abdul Nasser was president of Egypt he saw fit to lay down very stringent rules that a dancer had to observe if she valued her job. Dancers were not permitted to show the upper part of their legs; dancing on table tops was also prohibited; they had to cover their stomachs; they couldn't do floor work and were forbidden from making any "offensive movements" during the dance. He later relaxed some of these stringent rules. After his death things opened up considerably.

The Oriental dance played an important part in the days of the Pharaohs. In the Ottoman Empire the Oriental dancer was an integral part of the harem. Because of Muslim religous objections, dancing girls are still looked upon rather quizzically; however, they are gaining respectability. We hope that the popularity and respect for the dance will increase even more as time goes by. It's moving into some pretty nifty places these days, but we still have a long way to go to clean up the profession. In 1974, the New York Daily News had a picture of the then secretary of state, Henry Kissinger, observing navel maneuvers, as they put it. As I saw it; it was just a picture of an Oriental dancer being admired by a distinguished gentleman. In the 1840's Gustave Flaubert, the Frenchman, wrote extensively about the dance. One of my favorite paintings of an Oriental dancer is one called "Dance of the Almeh," done by Gérôme in 1863, which now graces the collection of the Dayton Art Institute in Ohio.

In 1893 Little Egypt and her dancing girls appeared at the Chicago World's Fair, and that's what started it all in the United States. Even with this fact, some scholars have their doubts. Some people say that Little Egypt never appeared there, but that the whole thing was a cunning feat by a clever agent.

There are definite regional styles of the Oriental dance being performed today, such as the Turkish, Persian, and Arabic styles, the latter giving birth to such folk dances as belledi, Berber, and so on. The Berbers, a North African tribe, developed quite early abdominal movements in their folk-culture dances. You can generally break down the Arab form of the dance into two parts: the classical and the danse du ventre, which has a folk quality and after which the Oriental dance has been patterned.

The Oriental dance is now going through what I'd like to term the "revival stage" here in America. It has its ups and downs. In the past few years a host of Oriental dance schools have cropped up all over the United States, as many people are realizing the physical benefits that can be derived from Oriental dancing. In the late 1950's Oriental dancers were an exclusive group and they were at quite a premium. Nowadays, everybody and his uncle is doing the danse orientale.

MAINTAINING DIGNITY

The Oriental dance is a very misunderstood dance form because many of the dancers who are performing are not aware of its history. Today, there are still Oriental dance teachers and performers who maintain a dignity and sense of history that are so important to the dance's survival. These studios are providing a fantastic and positive contribution to the women who have tuned into the exercise quality of the dance. On the other hand, there are some new Oriental dance studios that are putting the wrong emphasis on the dance, and I have every hope that we will weed out those who would interpret the dance as a sex-filled, bump and grind, jellied nothingness and nothing more.

The woman's body is a beautiful organism, and as such should be treated with respect at all times. Many professionals in the business think of the Oriental dance at times as a fertility dance (a preparation for childbirth), and indeed it could also be looked at as a celebration of birth. When a dancer performs this type of folkloric dance she usually starts with a happy-type melody which indicates the joy she is experiencing with a new human being growing within her, readying itself to confront the outside world. She then goes into a slow number which paints a picture of the pain that she is going through while the infant is announcing to her that it is ready to be born. Here, a good dancer will interpret the muscle contractions in the abdominal region of her body. Then for awhile she'll return to the up-tempo beat that expresses her joy. All of a sudden she'll writhe with pain again, oftentimes falling to the floor to seek solace—the contractions continue, and the dance takes on an ecstatically beautiful mood as we see our dancer happily engaged in the delivery of the child. After this she rejoices and dances vigorously with all the life and joy that she has left in her body. Thus one of the oldest dance forms known to man takes shape. The woman has expressed herself.

We have also learned that a woman at childbirth was entertained by women friends to keep her mind away from the pain she was suffering. She would imitate the contractions of her friends and thus ease her pain. This practice continues in many remote parts of the Middle East even today.

Many men also do this dance. We in the modern world often refer to the pains that some men go through when their wives are having a baby as "sympathy pains." Well, perhaps the men are expressing themselves too, as well as the closeness and oneness they feel with the woman when she is experiencing the birth of a child. In many Middle Eastern countries men dress in women's clothing to perform their dances.

I would only say "bravo" to the man who has that ability to express himself and his innermost feelings. In the kabuki dances of Japan, which were developed in the seventeenth century, both male and female roles were performed by male actors. If we go further back in history we will see that in many civilizations only men performed the dances, and that in many, women were frowned upon if they dared express themselves in this way. In Shakespeare's days, for example, women were not allowed on the stage. For this reason I would recommend my book to both men and women so that we can indeed get rid of some more of the stereotyped ideas that bind us into neatly labeled categories of male and female.

You know that old cliché, "Some of my best friends are . . .?" Well, some of my best friends are *male* Oriental dancers. I might also add that they are some of the finest dancers we have in the business today. Their physical condition inspires envy in many a male and female. Thanks to the dance they are able to maintain a graceful, healthy body.

TWO SCHOOLS OF ORIENTAL DANCING

There are basically two schools of Oriental dancing techniques alive and well in the United States today. One is the Turkish school and the other is the Arabic school. From these we have many other styles originating in a sort of eclectic Oriental dance form.

The Turkish and Arabic styles differ in that the rhythms are different. The basic character of Arabic music is the use of the quarter tone intervals. This makes the Arabic rhythm a bit strange to the American ear. Although some of these rhythms are different, they sometimes come together in a marriage that exudes harmony across cultural lines. Geographic boundaries are not recognized by the bright, lively, and exciting rhythms. The taksim is one of these rhythms. This is an improvised creative melody usually performed as an oud solo. The dancer uses this for her slow floor work.

The Turkish style of Oriental dancing is a very fluid style. The steps are wider than the Arabic steps, the body moves with larger movements, and the veil is used with much flourish and abandon. The Turkish karslimar or 9/8 rhythm is one of the more beautiful Turkish rhythms. The dancer uses this to inspire climactic joy in her routine.

The Arabic style as manifested in the cabaret style of Oriental dancing is rather bouncy with a kind of staccato rhythm. Even within the Arab world one notices regional differences. The dancer's steps are much smaller than in the Turkish style of dancing. Emphasis is placed on hip and foot movements. Shimmies, undulations, and an almost Indian approach to footwork is the order of the day in Arabic dancing. A great deal of controlled stomach movement is also visible. This style of dancing originated because the Bedouins and other Arab tribes did not have much room in which to dance, so they simply utilized the space they had.

Many folk dance steps have found their way into the Oriental dance. The Arabic debke is one of them. Arabic dancing also includes a vast variety of styles, such as the Egyptian, Algerian, Moroccan and Tunisian. These types of dances would be better known to the general public as folk dancing. Some of the more popular groups are the Ghawazees of Egypt, Gnaouas of Morocco, Berbers of North Africa, and the Ouled Nail of Algeria.

There are many other "props" that are utilized in the dance; for example, the sword and the cane. I have also witnessed a dancer using a snake in her act. Sword and cane dances are traditional Middle Eastern dances still performed today.

Listed here you'll find one record of each of the following categories of music: Arabic, Armenian, Greek, and Turkish styles. It is important for you to learn to differentiate between the various musical styles, so I would suggest that you make this initial investment to get you on your way.

1. **Arabic music:** *Belly Dance Music*, The Flames of Araby Orchestra, Vocals by George Abdo—Monitor
2. **Armenian music:** *Armenian Love Songs*, Roupen Altiparmakian—High Fidelity
3. **Greek music:** *The Feenjon Goes Greek*, Menachem Dworman—Monitor
4. **Turkish music:** *Alla Turca*, Ozel—El-Ay Records

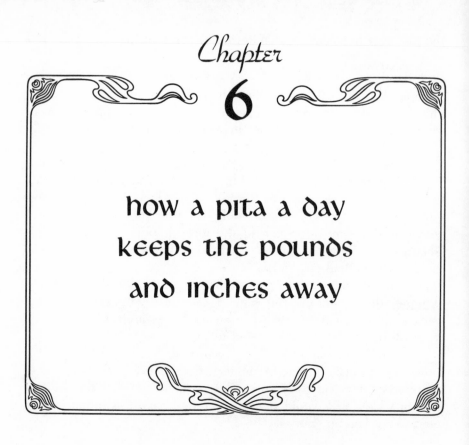

Chapter 6

how a pita a day keeps the pounds and inches away

The Arabs call their round bread "khubz" and the Greeks call it "pita." This type of bread became popular in New York when Greek souvlaki stands sprang up all over the city. The Greeks have adopted this bread for their gyros (hero sandwiches), doner kebabs, and souvlaki. They fill the round bread with delicacies and sell them in their fast-food stands. This sight has become very popular in the New York City area, but it is fast spreading to many other cities in the United States.

The natural color of the pita bread is that of a white bread; however, just the other day I saw some *whole-wheat* pita. This one has a few less calories than the regular pita bread, but at least now you have a choice to make. This whole-wheat pita is a bit too Americanized for my liking; however, this phenomenon shows that people are definitely becoming more and more aware of the health aspects of what they eat. It also shows that sooner or later foreign things in America always take on a little bit of America. There are even some major American bread companies now making their own versions of the Arabic bread. Whole-wheat pita has a lot of fiber in it, and that is excellent for you to incorporate into your eating habits.

Pita bread is very nutritious—it has proteins, thiamine, riboflavin, niacin, and iron. It is made with no oils or fats and it is low in calories. It is also one of the most versatile breads I know. It has a definite personality of its own. You can split it open and make little pizzas, you can use it for dips, you can pop it into your toaster and use your favorite spread on it, or you can use it as the Arabs do (I'll explain this later on). I have a girlfriend who stuffs her pita bread with caviar!

Albert T. didn't stuff his pita with caviar, but with hundreds of different nutritious goodies. Albert weighed 140 pounds before he began eating and exercising sensibly. He was about 15 pounds overweight for his medium frame. In only 3 weeks after starting his "pita bread diet," as he likes to call it, he showed a significant weight loss. He lost about 17 pounds during this time. His 5'2" petite self is a bundle of new-found energy.

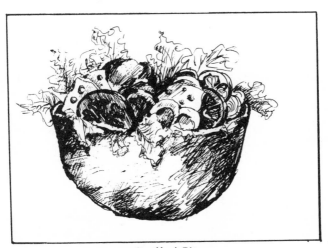

Stuffed Pita

THE VALUE OF BREAD

We read in the Bible that bread is the staff of life. Jesus performed miracles with bread. In St. Matthew, Chapter 15, Jesus feeds over four thousand people with seven loaves of bread and a few little fishes. In St. John, Chapter 6, he feeds five thousand men with five barley loaves and two fishes.

I relate these things to you, not because I want you to perform any miracles with bread, but to point out that from the time of Jesus bread played an important role in the lives of people. Jesus performed many miracles with bread as a symbol of life. In First Corinthians, we read of the bread they broke celebrating the communion of the body of Christ. Today in many religions this ritual is still celebrated using wafers and wine.

Bread plays an important part in many religions. For example, in Judaism there is the *shrewbread*, the twelve loaves of bread eaten every Sabbath. The shrewbread is placed on the table in the holy of holies of the Biblical tabernacle and the Temple in Jerusalem as an offering by the priests of God and eaten by them at the end of the week. Leviticus, Chapter 24, explains this ritual to us.

There are countless phrases using bread in them where bread means something different in each. Take for example the following:

1. Take the bread out of someone's mouth—take away the livelihood from someone.
2. Bread and butter—someone's livelihood.
3. Breadwinner—someone who earns a livelihood for himself and/or someone else.
4. Cast one's bread upon the waters—to act charitably.
5. Know on which side one's bread is buttered—to know which things are to your advantage.
6. Break bread—share your food with someone, a sharing as in the act of communion. This is a great Middle Eastern tradition which is practiced to show friendship.

BREAD AS A LUXURY

Even in the poorest of homes in cities and towns of the Middle East, bread is always on the table. Bread, black olives, and cheese are the staples of the poorer families. There are a few places, however, where bread is a bit scarce. For example, bread to the people of the desert (the Bedouins) is a luxury because there is little wheat there. They depend on fruit from the date palm, milk, and camel meat for their food. Other foods available to them are almonds, coffee, grapes, sugar cane, and watermelons.

When I was in Istanbul, Turkey, cheese had become very expensive and had to be cut out of the poorer families' eating pattern because of its prohibitive price. Then later on the olives started to go up in price and, of course, some people could not afford them either. Bread remained on the table—a lonely source of comfort. One thing about bread is that it can seemingly fill you up and give you a false sense of having eaten enough. If you eat only bread and nothing else you will suffer from severe malnutrition. In this rich society of ours, would you believe that there are still people who suffer from this condition? When things got better in Istanbul, then cheese and olives came back to the poor man's table. The olive was from ancient times an important item to the people of the Middle East, Greece, and Turkey. It provided them with light (oil burning in their lamps), cooking oil (great olive oil), and was even used as soap.

In my book I am not advocating that you follow a poor man's eating pattern by any means. I am just trying to show you the importance of bread in the eating habits of the people of the Middle East.

Of course there are many other cultures where bread is an integral part of every meal. Where would the Italians or the French be without their breads? *Mon dieu*! You walk on the streets of any Italian or French city and you see the people with their loaves of bread under their arms, in baskets, on their heads, and in all sorts of strange places. We in the United States are so unimaginative when it comes to carrying bread. I suppose that we should thank our technology for giving us plastic wrappings to keep undesirable germs off of bread and other things. As far as I am concerned, the lack of wrappings for the bread has left it open to the naked eye and therefore attached some sort of incredible sexiness to it. Think about it for a while, maybe you will see what I mean.

BREAD AS AN EATING UTENSIL

For the people of the Middle East, their bread becomes spoon, fork, and plate to them—bread is therefore a most important part of life. One reason for this is that expensive cutlery is not readily available—steel products are quite expensive in that part of the world. In the more affluent homes bread is still used in this manner; it's a part of their tradition even though silverware is on the table. Another reason that bread comes in handy is that a great many of the meals eaten are in liquid or semi-liquid form as soups, stews, and gravies. People of the Middle East do not eat big chunks of meat as we do here in the United States. Bread soaks up all of those gravies very nicely, and besides that, bread tastes so good dipped in just about anything. I remember joining my grandmother for her early morning coffee. My mother wouldn't let me drink coffee. "Too much caffein for a small child," she'd say. So I would have to sneak into my grandmother's room early in the morning when everyone was still asleep and she would dunk bread in her coffee and give it to me. Of course the forbidden nature of the whole procedure made it taste even better than it actually was. And, oh, did that coffee aroma get to me. Even today when I smell freshly brewed coffee I think of my grandmother.

In many parts of Morocco and other parts of the Middle East no utensils are used at all. This brings to mind one of the great Moroccan traditions—*couscous*. Couscous is like a finely cracked wheat, mixed with vegetables, lamb, or chicken. Moroccans eat this dish with their fingers. Some of the Moroccan restaurants that I have frequented will only give you utensils if you request them. Part of the fun of trying this dish is going the whole traditional route and eating it with your fingers. What better "utensil" to use? After all, fingers are always there when you need them. You don't have to go searching for them as I often have to do when I bring my lunch to school and for the life of me I can't find a fork anywhere.

You should be able to just dig in with your fingers. Of course they should be washed thoroughly before you do so. In the religion of Islam, people use their right hand to eat and their left hand to do other tasks. To the American way of life the idea of eating with the fingers is a messy business, but then just think of it, soap and water are readily available to us. After a meal the Moroccans will wipe their hands with a wet towel and sprinkle some rose water over them. Oh, what a lovely fragrance. This is even sprinkled over the whole body after the meal. It's a glorious tradition.

Couscous can also be used to make desserts. All you would have to do is mix in some raisins, currants, and some chopped almonds and cook it in your favorite fruit juice. This of course would be served cold.

Pita bread or *khubz* can be bought at most Middle Eastern stores, and even in some supermarkets. This points out the fact that more and more Americans are getting into the fun they can have with pita bread. I have been toying around with a certain philosophy for a long time, which is simply this: *A pita a day keeps the pounds away.* I am now going to share this with you. I use pita bread because it is so easy to stuff with all sorts of delicious things. It's not like regular bread that allows everything to ooze out of it before you get a chance to bite into it. How many times have you bitten into a tuna fish sandwich and had the tuna drip out all over the place? Pita bread is small, compact, and round and you can cut a small piece off the side, puff it open, and you're ready to have the time of your life stuffing goodies into it. This meal will also help your budget because most of the ingredients are relatively inexpensive, and then you can stuff the pita just so much and no more. Do not cheat and overstuff them. Furthermore, do not buy the large-size pita breads unless you are entertaining a lot of people. The small size, which is approximately five inches in diameter, should be the one you use. To cut down on the amount of ingredients you put in your pita bread, you can cut larger and larger pieces away until you have only half a pita to stuff. Another alternative would be to use the pita petites which are only about four inches in diameter.

BREAKING BREAD

Middle Easterners never cut the pita bread with a knife. Small pieces are always broken off and used to scoop up the food. This is such great fun. It's a great feeling of camaraderie to sit down with friends around a low table in front of a basket of pita bread and some hummus or whatever and to break bread and dip into the mix. No one needs individual plates. Everyone just digs into the one plate. Just think of all the dishes that you don't have to wash after the meal. After you try this you will throw away your crackers and potato chips.

Pita bread can be eaten fresh as you buy it or it can be warmed on a grill or in an oven. It should be eaten as soon as it is warmed, otherwise it tends to get hard. Middle Easterners never put butter on their bread, and neither should you. This surely helps to cut down on your cholesterol intake.

DISCOVERING NEW EATING PATTERNS

Now down to the business of what to do with the pita bread. May I suggest that you change your eating patterns for about two weeks, more if you wish, and see whether you can lose a few inches from around your waist? Instead of eating the same old cottage cheese and yogurt for lunch, fill your pita bread with some nutritious foods and eat just one pita for lunch. If you're having fun with this, have one for dinner too. Why not have a pita party? To do this all you have to do is make a lot of delicious "dips," stack up the pita bread, and you're ready to go. This can be one of the easiest parties you have ever thrown because, just think of it, there is no big cooking involved in a party like this and everybody can make their own pita sandwich. It will be up to you to provide a wide variety of "stuffings," and your guests can have a lot of fun experimenting with the various dishes. Now let's get back to the dinner table.

Before you start eating these delicacies, keep one fact in mind—counting calories is not enough to keep your weight down. You must demonstrate a great deal of control to change your eating pattern. When you do my exercises I ask you to prepare your mind and body for them. I am also going to ask you to prepare your mind and body before you eat. This will be a most difficult task, but you can do it, and in order to obtain results it is imperative that you bring a relaxed mind to your eating.

Clear your mind of all thoughts about food, emotional problems, and all the other things that clutter it up. Go a step further and clear your mind of everything. Relax your mind, relax your body. Some people say a little prayer to the Lord before they eat. I am convinced that this pause, when you close your eyes, helps you to relax as well as give praise to the Lord. It wouldn't be a bad idea if you did this also. After all, we should be thankful that we have been provided with food on our table. In the Bible, in Deuteronomy, Chapter 8, Verse 3, it tells us that "man doth not live by bread only, but by every word that proceedeth out of the mouth of the Lord does man live." In my interpretation of these words I find that he is attaching a great importance to bread, indeed to food in general. Of course the ultimate importance was His word. Not a bad idea.

Before you say your little prayer, remember to clear your mind completely and become calm and relaxed. Linger a moment. Find solace and peace in it. Spend at least five minutes "relaxing," but for heaven's sake don't fall asleep, although this may be thoroughly desirable because you could skip the meal altogether and lose a great deal more weight! Well, for those of you who are still awake and ready to eat, bon appetit!

In this chapter I have included some of the basic recipes that I have found to be appetizing and nutritious stuffings for the pita bread. Many of them are fun and kooky and really different. They may even seem improbable at first, but just try them; you'll change your mind. Let your imagination run wild and dream up some fancy recipes of your own. Just remember that you should not stuff too much into the pita bread because you would be defeating the whole idea of regulating your food intake. If the stuffing is oozing out all over the place, you have too much in the pita bread. I have found that about three-fourths of a cup of ingredients is just about right.

This idea of stuffing goodies into pita bread reminds me of two stories of some friends of mine. This idea changed a woman's entire life. Linda L., a comedienne who used to use her excess weight as the basis of her comedy routines, confessed to me after her show one night that her "extra set of hips" was hurting her career. She found there were more opportunities for slim comediennes. Linda said she had tried every diet but found them all to be "too routine." I suggested that she try my eating pattern and exercise plan for two weeks. The two weeks lasted for six months, and this newly trim comedienne is now doing T.V. commercials and at this writing has obtained a part in a movie. She said that her outlook on life has changed as much as her figure, and she wakes up each morning looking forward to the positive experience of each new day. When I asked what happened to her extra set of hips, she replied, "I put them in my pita bread and ate them." Goodbye fat for Linda!

Then there was Joan K., a mathematics teacher who was spending more time multiplying calories than dividing fractions. She began my eating pattern over the summer vacation. For two months she dispensed with her regular routine of counting calories and filled her pita bread instead of her stomach. Joan was delighted by the results. Calling to thank me, she said, "My midriff bulge has disintegrated. I have a waistline again, a waistline that is a pleasure to measure."

My eating pattern doesn't advocate eating bread alone, but this pita bread idea is, shall we say, a way of wrapping up all your nutrients in a neat little package. The idea is to eat a well-balanced, nutritious meal.

In Isaiah, Chapter 55, Verse 2, we are warned to "eat ye that which is good," and it goes on to say, "and let your soul delight in fatness." That last part gave me a chuckle. I bet that in those days no one worried about their eating pattern. One reason, I suppose, was that life was so simple and they didn't have to worry about cyclamates and all sorts of additives to their food. Unfortunately, things are no longer that simple for us and we have to ferret out all the impurities in our foods.

One of the truly profound passages in the Bible is Revelations, Chapter 2, Verse 7, "He that hath an ear, let him hear what the Spirit saith unto the churches; to him that overcometh will I give to eat of the tree of life, which is in the midst of the paradise of God." I am by no means preaching religion here; however, I think that this could serve as a good motto by which to live your life—"eat of the tree of life." Live your life to the fullest, never regretting a moment of it, never looking back, just looking ahead to each new happening with zest and vitality.

Pita Recipes

1. Pita-burger

Take a handful of chopped lean meat.

Season with salt, pepper, and thyme to taste.

Make a flat pattie and broil until cooked.

Stuff into pita bread with some diced tomato and diced pickle.

2. Anchovy Pita

Mix the following ingredients together:

1 small can anchovies

½ cup mozzarella cheese (grated)

6 cherry tomatoes (sliced)

3 black pitted olives (chopped finely)

Stuff into pita bread.

3. Asparagus Pita

Spread 2 tablespoons mayonnaise in pita bread.

Add about 6 asparagus spears.

4. Avocado Pita

Mash ½ of a small avocado with 1 teaspoon of mayonnaise.

Add salt and pepper to taste.

Add 1 slice of raw onion (optional).

Stuff into pita bread.

5. Baba Ghannouj Pita

Follow my recipe for baba ghannouj (eggplant dip).

Stuff 4 tablespoons of it into pita bread.

6. Cheese Pita

Take a few slices of Greek feta cheese.

Add 2 slices of tomato.

Salt and pepper to taste.

Stuff into pita bread.

7. Chicken Liver Pita

Boil about 4 chicken livers until cooked (about 10 minutes) and then mash them with a little of the broth.

Add 1 slice of finely chopped onion.

Salt and pepper to taste.

Stuff into pita bread.

8. Cottage Cheese Pita

Mix together the following ingredients:

1 cup cottage cheese

3 asparagus spears

3 radishes (sliced)

Stuff into pita bread.

9. Cucumber Pita

Mix together the following ingredients:

½ cucumber, peeled and cut in slices

1 scallion, finely chopped

¼ teaspoon fresh mint (⅛ teaspoon if dried)

¼ teaspoon fresh parsley (⅛ teaspoon if dried)

⅛ teaspoon thyme

Salt and pepper to taste.

Stuff into pita bread.

10. Cucumber-Yogurt Pita

Mix together the following ingredients:

½ cucumber, peeled and finely chopped

⅛ teaspoon garlic powder

⅛ teaspoon dried mint

¼ cup yogurt

Salt and pepper to taste

Stuff into pita bread.

11. Egg Pita

Take 2 eggs and do what you will with them. Follow my recipe for onion eggs or spinach eggs if you wish.

Stuff into pita bread.

12. Eggplant Pita

Take 1 medium eggplant, peel off the skin, and slice into ¼ inch slices.

Add salt and let stand until beads of water appear.

Soak up the water with a paper towel.

Fry in oil until brown, drain on paper towel.

Stuff 4 or 5 slices into pita bread with 4 tablespoons of plain yogurt.

You can eat this either hot or cold.

13. Fish Pita

You can use just about any cooked fish (avoid fried fish). Please remove the bones before putting it in the pita bread.

Salt and pepper to taste.

Stuff into pita bread.

14. Green Pepper Pita

Chop finely 1 medium green pepper, 1 small onion, and 1 small tomato.

Sauté in 1 tablespoon safflower oil.

Add ¼ cup whipped low-fat cottage cheese.

Stuff into pita bread.

Sprinkle inside with 1 tablespoon grated mozzarella cheese.

Put pita bread in oven until mozzarella cheese melts.

Top with shredded lettuce.

15. Health Salad Pita

Mix the following ingredients together:

¼ green pepper, finely chopped.

¼ cup shredded red cabbage.

¼ cup shredded lettuce.

3 black olives, pitted and finely chopped.

1 scallion, chopped finely.

2 slices tomato, chopped finely.

¼ carrot, grated.

1 slice mozzarella cheese finely chopped.

1 slice feta cheese.

1 teaspoon fresh bean sprouts.

1 teaspoon olive oil.

1 teaspoon wine vinegar.

dash of garlic powder.

dash of oregano.

Salt and pepper to taste.

Mix all ingredients together, top with 3 tablespoons hummus (see recipe).

Stuff into pita bread.

This is going to be like your "Dagwood" sandwich, chock full of nutrients. This one you can allow to overflow a little.

16. Hummus Pita

Follow my recipe for chick pea dip.

Stuff 4 tablespoons of hummus into pita bread.

Middle Eastern people usually use the pita bread to dip up the spread; however, for our purposes, because we want to control the amount of things you put into the pita, we want you to fill your pita bread with a specified amount of the spread at this point. Sometimes I also sneak a hamburger in with the hummus, and is this ever delicious!

17. Peach Pita

Cut one large fresh peach in slices.

Add 2 tablespoons of sour cream or yogurt.

Mix together.

Stuff into pita bread.

18. Pear Pita

Cut one fresh pear in slices.

Add 2 tablespoons of sour cream or yogurt.

Mix together.

Stuff into pita bread.

19. Salmon Pita

Take a small can of salmon.

Add 1 scallion, finely chopped.

Mix in 1 tablespoon of oil and 1 tablespoon of lemon juice.
Add 1 tablespoon mayonnaise.
Stuff into pita bread.

20. Soybean Pita

Take 2 cups soybeans.
Place in 3 quarts water and soak overnight.
Add 1 tablespoon polyunsaturated oil.
Add 1 small onion, 1 small tomato, 1 stalk celery, finely chopped.
Salt and pepper to taste.
Boil for about 5 hours until soybeans are soft and all water is absorbed.
Take 4 tablespoons of this mixture and stuff into pita bread.

21. Spinach and Egg Pita

Take ½ cup of cooked spinach and one hard-boiled egg, chopped.
Add 2 tablespoons of sour cream or plain yogurt.
Sprinkle some grated cheese (any kind) on this mixture.
Stuff into pita bread.

22. Tomato-Onion Pita

Chop 1 medium tomato into cubes.
Add one slice of onion, chopped.
Add 1 teaspoon oil, ½ teaspoon lemon juice, a sprinkle of garlic powder, and ⅛ teaspoon dried mint.
Salt and pepper to taste.
Stuff into pita bread.

23. Tongue Pita

Follow your favorite recipe for cooking tongue.
Cut about 4 slices.
Spread some mayonnaise and mustard inside the pita bread.
Stuff tongue into pita bread.

24. Tuna Pita

Take 1 small can tuna.

Mix with 1 tablespoon of mayonnaise.

Stuff into pita bread.

An alternative would be to follow the recipe for salmon pita.

25. Tuna and Cucumber Pita

Take 1 small can tuna.

Mix with ½ cucumber, finely chopped.

Add 1 tablespoon chives.

Salt and pepper to taste.

Stuff into pita bread.

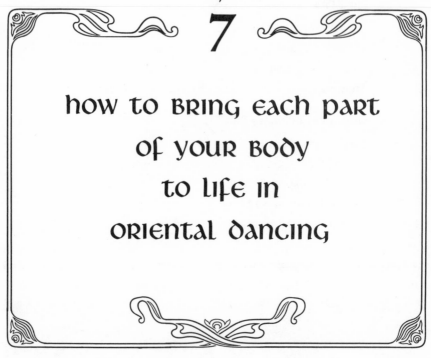

how to bring each part of your body to life in oriental dancing

I'm a public school teacher as well as an Oriental dancer, but I learned less about taking care of my body in teacher education than in Oriental dancing. My night-time career is what started me on a pattern of regular exercise and watching my diet. Before I started dancing, I would eat anything and everything that came down the turnpike! During my whole childhood, no one, at home or at school, instilled any facts of nutrition in me, and no one recommended that I exercise. In college, I only took physical education because it was required. I also had a class in health education, and picked up some valuable information, but I never got any feeling that it was really necessary for life outside class. Once the class was over I felt it was all right for me to go back to my old evil ways, eating poorly and never exercising. Regretfully, nobody tried to teach me to take care of my body on an ongoing basis.

My awareness of my own body increased when I became a dancer, because I realized I needed an attractive figure. In order to get Oriental dancing jobs I had to look good, even though nobody cared what might be wrong inside my body. But I began to get interested in having a healthy body as well as an attractive one. Slowly, but surely, I began to read about bodily health. The more health books and articles I read, the more all the shocking revelations about "junk foods" turned me toward healthier foods.

During this same time, I was learning to exercise, doing regular Oriental dance exercises, and felt the need for nutritious foods. I set a new goal of having an inward beauty as well as an outward beauty. This has been my goal for many, many years now, and I hope it will become your goal too.

As a professional Oriental dancer, I am constantly approached by people who ask me, "How do you stay in such great shape?" Of course, before the question even comes out, they think of an answer and add, "Oh, the Oriental dancing keeps you in shape, doesn't it?" My reaction is just to say "Yes, it does," and let it go at that. Over the years, though, I've given much thought to those two questions and have finally come up with a better explanation of why I "stay in shape."

Yes, Oriental dancing does help—the exercise value is built into the dance. However, I have to watch what I eat, too. It's great to participate in such a fun-filled activity that makes you lose pounds and inches while you do it, but it's a strenuous activity that requires good nutrition.

Many people who see me dance don't realize the amount of energy I expend during a performance. They look at a dancer going through her routine and think it looks so easy. Let me clear up that misconception right here and now. It takes a great deal of energy and stamina to perform for from twenty to thirty minutes on stage. I use every muscle of my body during a performance, and of course the bright, hot lights make me perspire, so I lose excess water. Even my mind is exercised because of my preoccupation with pleasing my audience. My body requires good nutrition to supply new energy.

Some so-called Oriental dancers may take it easy and "fake it," but they don't last. It takes years of study and work to perfect this art, and the public won't accept phonies for very long. Such dancers may briefly give the illusion of being professionals, but that will last for a very short while because they can only fool the people so long and no longer. You can't develop the much needed strength in your muscles and body if you do not approach the dance with the diligence and dedication that your body and the dance deserve.

AFTER THE DANCE

After the dance your body feels a momentary exhaustion, but that lasts for only a little while, and before you know it you could go on for another twenty minute performance. The dance leaves you in a state of ecstasy, you get "high" from your performance. Your body tingles. You feel reborn. (Through my exercises you are going to achieve this feeling too!)

It isn't necessary for you to perform every single night in order to stay trim, although that would be one way of doing it. Actually, I do not perform every night; however, what I do is supplement my performances with the Oriental dance exercises I have described in this book. From time to time I also get involved with other dance forms. When you have mastered the exercises, you too can start "performing" for your friends and relatives. If you become truly interested in extending your experience, who knows, you too may go on to become a professional dancer.

Many of the exercises that are included here are movements that are found in gymnastics. Combined together in the proper way they make up one of the loveliest dance forms in the world—the Oriental dance (belly dance, danse orientale, or as the Turks call it, "gobek atmak"—throwing the navel or belly). The form that these exercises take makes it a very pleasant way to lose weight, and I assure you that you will improve the quality of your life.

Take the case of some friends of mine who live in Florida.

"Auntie" L. was half of a retired couple whom I had met while vacationing in Florida. We got to talking on the beach one day, and of course she found out about my Oriental dancing career. I can't talk to anyone for five minutes without bringing up the subject of good health and exercise.

She had been looking for something interesting to do, and I thought that this was the perfect thing for her. I also explained to her about the variety in the Middle Eastern kitchen.

After visiting a Greek restaurant with her she was "hooked." One year later she is now giving free group Oriental dance lessons and her whole retirement village is benefiting. Incidentally, she corresponds with me and tells me that she feels 20 years younger and is keeping extra weight off with her weekly classes.

Her husband likes her new hobby and now calls her "my sexy belly dancer." "Auntie" L. also tells me that her sex life has improved greatly. I always tease her and say, "At your age, Auntie L, you should be doing more housework and less fooling around."

I will make no attempt here to give a quick and easy way to be a professional Oriental dancer because you cannot become one by reading a book. One needs the personal contact of a good teacher and years of long hard work to become a performer. It's like trying to make love from a manual, it just cannot be done with any real satisfaction. In this book I have included many exercises that I have done over the years and continue to do in order to "stay in shape." You will also get a flavor and a feel for the culture surrounding the dance. This chapter deals with the physical value derived from the exercises. The Oriental dance exercises are a lot of fun and will keep your body in trim.

REGIONAL VARIATIONS

The exercises included here are some of the simpler steps we Oriental dancers use during a performance. Some of the specialty dances you will see the dancers perform today include the following: the Oriental dance, classical or cabaret style; the belledi; the dance of the seven veils; dances of the Ghawazi; the Zar; the Guedra or trance dance of Morocco; the dances of the Ouled Nail, a North African nomadic tribe; the Pharaonic dance; the sword dance and the Egyptian cane dance (Raks Al-Assaya); the Raqs-es-saif, a dance of balance and skill; the Nahl, which is filled with mimetic gestures. These dances come from different parts of the Middle East and are mainly regional dances. They take the form of chain dances, combat dances, improvisational dances, religious dances, and the one most popular in the United States—the Oriental dance. In several regions many of the dances are done accompanied only by hand clapping, drums, and rhythm instruments, either in isolation or in any combination of the three forms. In the more sophisticated and modern nightclubs of today one sees electric guitars and other instruments being used to make up some rather elaborate orchestras. For example, in Cairo, Egypt, it's nothing to see a sixteen-piece orchestra accompany a dancer.

The Oriental dance runs into a great deal of trouble because the more orthodox religious teachings of Islam do not permit music or dance. Even today, in many Middle Eastern countries so-called "nice girls" are never seen dancing in public. The Oriental dance and other dance forms cannot be justified by a devout believer in the teachings of Islam. The scantiness of costume used in the Oriental dance, the music associated with it, and the drinking of alcoholic beverages that takes place in the clubs where the dance is performed are a few of the reasons orthodox Muslims object to it. Most people in the Middle East do not interpret their religious rules quite so strictly. In Egypt there are some first-class Oriental dancers who are highly respected. There, a wedding wouldn't be a wedding if at least two Oriental dancers didn't perform.

THE WHIRLING DERVISHES

The same discrimination is seen against the Whirling Dervishes or Mevleni of Turkey even today. For example, they would never refer to what they do as dancing. In the past they "did their thing" under the guise of a religious outpouring. They would chant prayers and work themselves up progressively by whirling around and around to a fevered pitch of a kind of trance dance. The Koran does not condone the use of music or dance, and so they had to *perform* in secret. Like everything else, today the Dervishes are gradually coming out of their secretiveness and are more openly performing their ancient ritual. You can see them perform today if you visit Konya in Turkey. A group even performed in the United States some time ago.

I recently finished reading a book on the Whirling Dervishes by Ira Friedlander, and I thought I'd include a few excerpts from his work to give you a better understanding of this ancient ritual. He tells us:

> The Mevleni order of Sufis known as the Whirling Dervishes began around 1258 in Konya, Turkey . . . They empty their hearts of all but the thought of God and whirl in the ecstatic movement of His breath . . . The Sema (whirling dance) of the dervishes is an expression of the cosmic joy experienced by the simultaneous effect of annihilation and glorification . . . The sikke, the tall honey-colored felt hat, represents the tombstone of man! . . . The Tennure (long white skirt) represents the shroud, and the khirqa (black cloak with long, large sleeves) symbolized the tomb. Beneath the cloak the turner wears a dasta gul (literally, a bouquet of roses) and a white jacket, the right side of which is tied down, the left hangs open. Around his waist is fastened the alif-lam-and (girdle of cloth about four fingers wide and two and a half feet long). On his feet are soft leather slippers which are ankle high . . . The ceremony is accompanied by a chorus that chants and by musicians. In 1925, Law 677 was intro-

duced into the Turkish Republic. It prohibited the procedure of initiation in the Whirling Dervishes. Twenty eight years later Sadettin Heper approached the mayor of Konya to make arrangements for the Mevlenis to whirl again. In December 1953, an audience was invited to the local cinema in Konya to see the Mevleni sema. Today the Mevlenis whirl their sacred dance each December in Konya accompanied by singer, the ney, kudum (drum) and rebab.*

I tell you all this because it will further help you to get into the feeling of all that this part of the world has to offer. In my book I deal with the Oriental dance, but you can go even further and try some of the other folk dances.

These "dance steps" or exercises, as I choose to call them for the purposes of this book, are called by various names by different performers. However, I have taken the consensus from a number of dancers and I have called these exercises by their most commonly known names. If you are going to do Oriental dance exercises then it behooves you to use some of the language that we dancers use. One of the problems we have in this dance field is that many dancers, instead of striving to bring the art to a high professional level and present some sort of coordinated effort, tend to isolate themselves in their own little world and the art then becomes splattered into little fragmented pieces. This is a very destructive path to follow. I have seen books appear where all sorts of fancy names are attached to these steps. I think that there should be much more cohesiveness between dancers so that we can further legitimize our art form. After all, in the ballet world, a *plié* is a *plié*, a *jeté* is a *jeté*, and a *battement* is a *battement*. I hope that in my lifetime I will see a great deal more coordinated effort taking place so that our "divisions" won't conquer us but that we will find some way to unite and become strong. One way of course would be to have some form of stabilized, universal categories for the dance steps used in the dance.

There are many aspects to the dance that I have chosen to omit from this book. I have not included any instruction for the use of the veil, that thin piece of flowing fabric that is such a beautiful, ethereal part of a dancer's routine. I have also not included any zill (finger cymbal) instruction because the main thing that I have culled from the Oriental dance for this book is the exercise aspect of the dance rather than teaching you all aspects of the dance. Actually, zill work could strengthen your hand muscles, but the intricacy of the teaching of that could fill another book so I chose to omit this.

The Whirling Dervishes by Ira Friedlander, with contributions by Nezih Uzel. (Copyright © 1975 by Ira Friedlander.)

I will be isolating various parts of the body and working to develop them because, as I said before, I am not teaching you how to do the Oriental dance, but rather giving you the benefit of my exercises to tone up your body and keep it working the way it should. I want your body to be stimulated physically and psychologically. My exercises are geared towards disciplining the body and the mind, getting the body into shape, and making you a more sensuous person. These exercises will also help in working out your aggressions, and this alone is worth a few minutes a day.

You must prepare yourself mentally before you start any of my exercises. Bring a positive mind to the exercises that will transport you to faraway exotic places you have always dreamed of visiting.

WHAT TO WEAR

Leotards and tights will do fine for your exercise outfit, but I would like you to go a step further and actually try to picture yourself as one of the ladies in the Sultan's harem and dress accordingly. For the men who pick up this book, go ahead and picture yourself as the sultan! In order to really get in the mood you can make yourself some sort of Middle Eastern outfit. Make sure that the outfit is comfortable as well as attractive. In Chapter 10 I have given you some directions on making a practice costume. The exercise costumes you see pictured in the exercises will also give you some ideas.

Start each exercise standing tall, buttocks tucked under, shoulders back, and stomachs in and "smile," as the Hawaiians say, "It no going broke your face." There is nothing more beautiful than a lovely smile on a dancer's face. Do the Oriental dance exercises for fifteen minutes *every day* if you are trying to lose weight. You must do your mind and body preparedness exercises before every exercise session. Do one exercise from each section until you master it then proceed to the next one. When you have learned all the exercises, then you can go back and choose one from each section to do every day. Remember to do your body stretches or other warm-up exercises first to limber up.

DANCING AWAY YOUR TROUBLES

Many people complain of symptoms directly stemming from anxiety or stress. My answer would be to dance your anxiety away. When you do the Oriental dance you are transported to another world—sensuous and abundantly rich with delicious intrigue. Although the dance will have a great influence on your being, you'll find that *you* can have an influence over it too. You should make it work for you. Impose your wishes, desires, and dreams on the dance. I have often used the dance to transport me in my imagination to an ancient Middle Eastern or Turkish palace where I become the Sultan's favorite dancing girl. It makes me feel like a woman all over. Try it, you'll like it! If this doesn't do wonders for your ego, I don't know what will. By the way, it will do a lot for your favorite man's ego too.

Why don't you try making your husband or loved one the Sultan? There is no need to travel to faraway shores. Your sultan can be found right there in your home. For the ladies who do not have one within easy reach, go out and get one quickly. Smother him with the riches only a sultan can afford. You'll maintain a svelte figure keeping him busy.

Instead of allowing your body to undergo stress or anxiety caused whenever a threatening or challenging event occurs, overcome this problem by getting involved with the Oriental dance. Instead of becoming addicted to drugs that control stress-induced anxiety, turn on to the danse orientale.

Oriental dancing can give you a whole new life as it did for Mary R., a lovely 57-year-old woman. After her husband died rather suddenly she was completely broken up over his death. To drown her sorrow, she turned to liquor and also tried to eat her unhappiness away. I met her when she was literally an overblown balloon, 35 pounds overweight. I felt it my duty to try to help her out of this miserable condition.

I knew that she was quite attractive before this tragedy occurred because she had shown me some of her pictures. After I gained her confidence, the first thing I tried to "wean" her from was the liquor. After all, she despised liquor when her husband was alive, so, although it was a challenge for me, I knew that given the right circumstances she would snap out of this suicidal course. I personally started to teach her some Oriental dance exercises and got her very involved in the Middle Eastern culture. My feeling was that she had a tremendous void to fill and I felt that I had the perfect thing with which to fill it.

She started to lose weight rather rapidly, and within a month she was a new person. Age does not limit participation in the Oriental dance, or for that matter, in a healthy eating pattern. She is not the only "older" woman that I have seen involved in this ancient art form. I think one of the main reasons for this is that you do not need a partner with which to enjoy the dance.

Mary needed this chance to freely express herself, and she didn't have to feel guilty that she didn't have a "partner." These days she's her attractive old self, full of vim and vitality and enjoying her life to its fullest extent minus the 35 excess pounds of sorrow.

Meditation has long provided an answer to this stress problem; however, I find that by itself meditation is too passive for my taste. Meditation is successful when you are able to concentrate for long periods of time. Besides that there is no *fun* in meditation. I am therefore suggesting that you use this concept when you do your Oriental dance exercises or when you eat, but go a step further and put a little fun in your life. If the body is relaxed and your attention is focused on your activity, be it exercise or eating, your body will be much more receptive to both. If you are tense and anxious you'll do more harm than good to your bodily functions.

Physicians tell us constantly that eating while you are excited tends to cause all sorts of problems. You must get turned on to the specific areas in your body and keep them well fed and well exercised. Your body deserves a lot of respect.

All of my Oriental dance exercises must be done to music, because music is an integral part of the mood you create. Without music, I believe that our lives would be null and void. Music doth soothe the spirit, and through the spirit the body is revitalized and inspired to perform the way it should.

You will need two basic tempos for these exercises—slow and fast. In the appendix you will find a list of some slow tunes and some fast tunes pulled from various records for your convenience. I have also included a very extensive list of Middle Eastern records for you to browse through. The more records you acquire, the more familiar you will become with the mood that is set by them. I have also included a list of record stores where you can find them. With the new popularity of the dance, many records can also be found in the regular record shops.

When you do your exercises, after each one relax your body, take a few deep breaths, inhale, exhale, and relax for a moment. You should not rush through your exercises, you should savor every moment of them.

MOVING VARIOUS BODY AREAS

I have started off with head exercises and worked my way through all the different sections of the body. Basically I have tried to simplify the exercises as much as possible because I know the actual pain that I have gone through trying to decipher complicated exercises while doing them from a book. The exercises are grouped for different areas of the body so that you can locate them easily.

When you see a good Oriental dancer perform you will notice that most of the movements are done in isolation. Movements are created for each individual part of the body. For variety, however, there are times when all parts of the body are used at the same time. This is usually done towards the end of certain segments of the dance, with particular emphasis on the finale, which should be a fantastic show of climactic ecstasy.

These Oriental dance exercises are exercises you can enjoy because they are done to music and they are flowing movements. You don't jerk your body parts in hastily contrived movements—you slowly and gracefully make patterns in space with your head, shoulders, waist, and so on.

They are not done in a vacuum known as "exercise." They are related to a culture that has been around for hundreds of years. They are an integral part of a people—an ancient people. So when you do the exercises it's very easy for your mind to transport you to the origins of the dance.

When you master the simpler exercises associated with the dance, then the possibilities are endless. You can carry them a step further and begin to learn some variations, and then start grouping certain ones together and amuse yourself.

SETTING REALISTIC GOALS

There is no point to setting impossible goals for yourself because that will only lead to frustrations. Try to set realistic goals for yourself. Try to set a goal of a loss of three to four pounds per week. If you need to lose a lot of weight then it will just take you a little longer to achieve your goal. There is no hurry. Haste will make waste, because if you try to starve yourself and do too much exercise you'll reach the point where you will begin to get overly hungry and overeat, and also skip days of exercise and start sliding back to your original weight. The steadier your exercise and eating pattern is, the more benefits you'll derive over a longer period of time.

Before you start your exercises you could warm up with a steady, rhythmic repetitive activity such as jogging, walking in place, or rope jumping so that you do not overtax your heart and circulation. These kinds of exercise will promote endurance by increasing your oxygen absorption capacity. This will be gradually increased over a period of time, and you'll be able to do more and more exercises for a longer period of time without getting tired. You can also use the body stretches to warm up, or the Sun Salutation yoga asana. By the same token don't abruptly stop your exercises. You'll feel dizzy or nauseated if you do. You must avoid this under all circumstances. Remember, exercises should be moderate in the beginning, and gradually increased as you progress.

The following deserves repeating as the correct posture for all exercises:

1. Head straight up, chin tucked in.
2. Shoulders straight.
3. Breast bone up.
4. Pelvis straight under trunk.
5. Knees bent slightly.
6. Feet slightly apart.
7. Hands at side.
8. Your position should be one of ease; do not strain.

For your convenience I've prepared a little chart of exactly what exercises you will be doing depending on whether you will be losing weight or maintaining your weight.

Maintaining Your Weight

Morning—5-10 minutes body stretches or other miscellaneous
exercises or the Sun Salutation yoga asana
15 minutes Oriental dance exercises

Evening—Every other day, all the body stretches or 10 minutes
other miscellaneous exercises
10 minutes water exercises every day.

Losing Weight

Morning—5-10 minutes body stretches or other miscellaneous
exercises or the Sun Salutation yoga asana

15 minutes Oriental dance exercises

Evening—Every day, all of the body stretches or 20 minutes other
miscellaneous exercises

15 minutes water exercises every day

Circular Head Slides

- Assume correct posture.
- Place both arms up directly over your head.
- Place the palms of your hands together.
- Slide your head over to the inside of the left elbow.
- Slide your head forward, sticking your chin out front as far as
you can.
- Slowly slide your head over to the inside of the right elbow.
- Slide your head back, tucking your chin into your neck.
- Slide your head over to the inside of the left elbow to complete
the circle.
- Return to the starting position.
- The head has made a complete circle.
- Repeat circular motion 4 times.

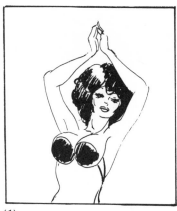

(1)

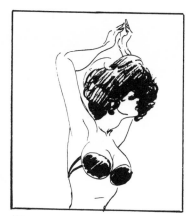

(2)

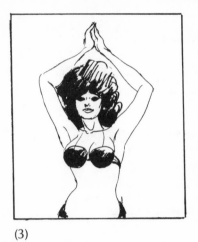 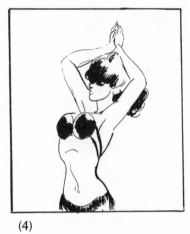

(3)   (4)

Circular Head Slides

Fast Shoulder Thrusts or Pushes

- Assume correct posture.
- Hands down at sides.
- Face forward, keeping shoulders straight.
- Thrust left shoulder forward.
- Return to starting position.
- Thrust right shoulder forward.
- Return to starting position.
- Alternate shoulders.
- Do this quickly without pausing, shoulders will vibrate.
- Repeat this exercise for about 1 minute.

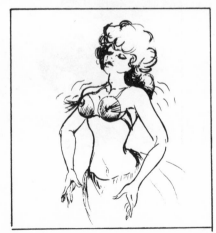

Fast Shoulder Thrusts or Pushes

Shoulder Circles

- Assume correct posture.
- Hands down at your sides.
- Thrust left shoulder forward slowly.
- Raise shoulder upward as far as you can—shoulder should almost touch your ear.
- Pull shoulder back and down to make a complete circle.
- Repeat 3 times.
- Thrust right shoulder forward slowly.
- Raise shoulder forward as far as you can—shoulder should almost touch your ear.
- Pull shoulder back and down to make a complete circle.
- Repeat 3 times.
- After alternating shoulders, do both shoulders together.
- Repeat 3 times.
  Feels good, yes?

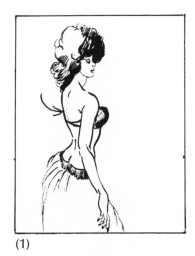

(1)

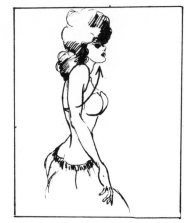

(2)

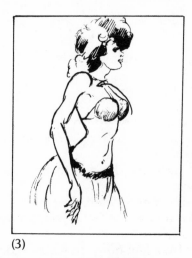

(3)

Shoulder Circles

Serpent Arms—Sidewards

- Assume correct posture.
- Arms straight down at sides.
- Bring left arm up slowly by your side.
- Lead with the elbow.
- Brush the side of your thigh with the palm of your hand as you raise it.

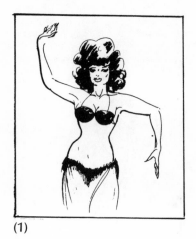
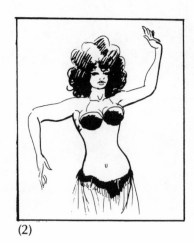

(1)   (2)

Serpent Arms

- Palm should be facing down.
- When your elbow reaches shoulder level, twist wrist and turn palm to face outwards with fingers facing towards the ceiling.
- Turn elbow downwards and start lowering left arm.
- Repeat 3 times.
- Do the same with the right arm.
- Repeat 3 times.
- Then alternate arms. The left arm should be going up when the right arm is coming down.
- Repeat 5 times.

Double Arm Circles

- Assume correct posture.
- Start with arms at your sides.
- Bring arms in front of your stomach.
- Slowly raise both arms up to shoulder level.
- Continue raising arms until they are over your head forming an arch.
- Palms should come together above the head. Lower arms in front of your face, still keeping palms fairly close together.
- When your hands reach the stomach, start raising them again.
- Continue circles slowly.
- Make sure arms cross each other in front.
- Repeat 5 times.

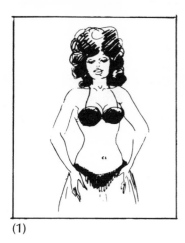

(1)

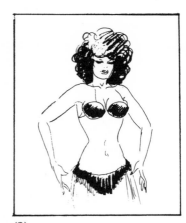

(2)

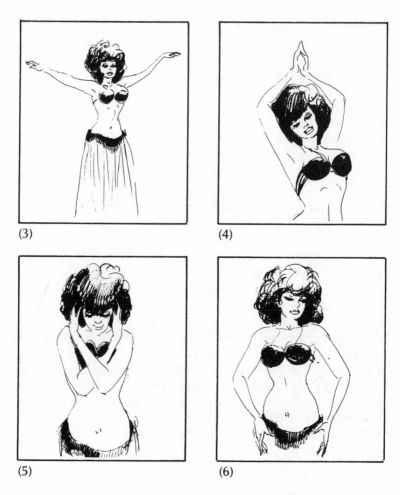

(3)

(4)

(5)

(6)

Double Arm Circles

Parallel Arm Circles

- Assume correct posture.
- Head straight.
- Start with arms at your sides.
- Slowly swing both arms to the left side.
- Continue up until they reach shoulder level.
- Continue up until they are above the head.
- Swing them over to the right and lower to starting position.
- You will have made a complete circle.

- Keep the arms as close together as possible so that they move almost as one.
- Repeat 5 times.

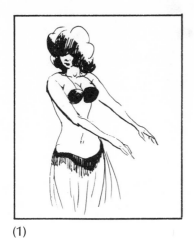

(1)

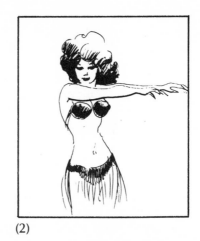

(2)

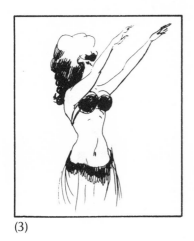

(3)

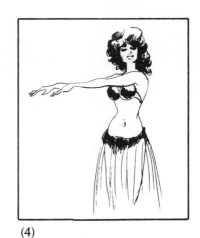

(4)

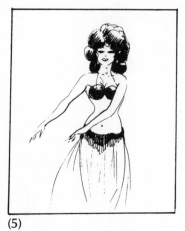

(5)

Parallel Arm Circles

Torso or Rib Circles

- Assume correct posture.
- Hands on hips.
- Lower body should be perfectly still.
- Slide rib cage from the waist over to the left side.
- Pull rib cage towards the back.
- Suck stomach in.
- Slide rib cage over to the right.
- Push rib cage out in front.
- Continue in a circular motion for about 2 minutes.

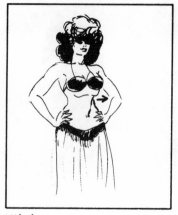

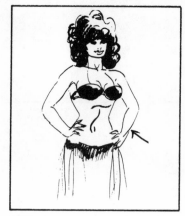

(1)left   (2)in

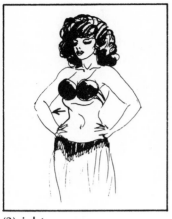 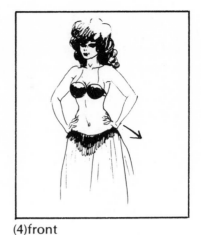

(3)right   (4)front

Torso or Rib Circles

Knee Bend and Rise

- Assume correct posture.
- Stand with feet slightly apart.
- Right foot in front of left foot.
- Hands out to the sides.
- Slowly lift your heels off the floor.
- Bend knees and descend to the floor.
- Keep upper torso erect, looking straight ahead.

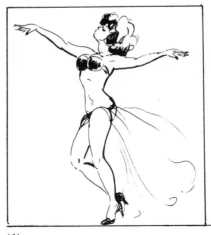

(1)

- As you descend, lower hands to the floor.
- Descend on both knees.
- To rise, bring left foot up in front of right foot.
- Place your weight on the left foot, push up with the right foot.
- Bring arms up at your side to shoulder level.
- Lower arms to your sides.
- Repeat 3 times.

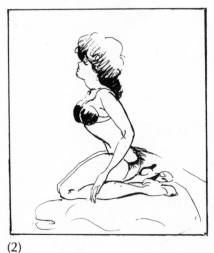
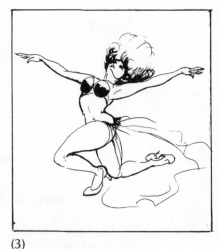

(2)   (3)

Knee Bend and Rise

Knee Pivots

- Assume correct posture.
- Stand with feet slightly apart.
- Right foot in front of left foot.
- Arms out to the sides.
- Slowly lift your heels off the floor.
- Bend knees and descend to the floor slowly.
- Kneel on both knees slowly.
- Bring left knee up, right knee remains on floor.
- Pivot on your right knee; this movement is achieved by moving the left foot around in a circle.
- Move foot to the left, counterclockwise, about 6 inches at a time.
- Make 2 complete circles.
- Lower left foot.
- Raise right foot and do the pivot clockwise.

- Make 2 complete circles.
- Each time you do this exercise try to pivot a little faster.

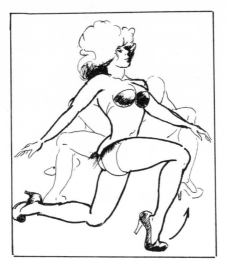

Knee Pivots

Knee Walk

- Assume correct posture.
- Stand with feet slightly apart.
- Right foot in front of left foot.
- Arms out to the sides.
- Slowly lift your heels off the floor.
- Bend knees slowly and descend to the floor.
- Kneel on both knees.
- Raise left knee up off floor.
- Put left foot on the floor.
- Pull right knee along the floor until it touches the left heel.
- Move left foot forward about one foot.
- Lower left knee to the floor.
- Raise right knee off the floor.
- Put right foot flat on the floor.
- Pull left knee along the floor ,until it touches the right heel.
- Continue for about 2 minutes.

This "walk" can be done in a straight line, in circles, or in any pattern you wish. The idea is to keep moving.

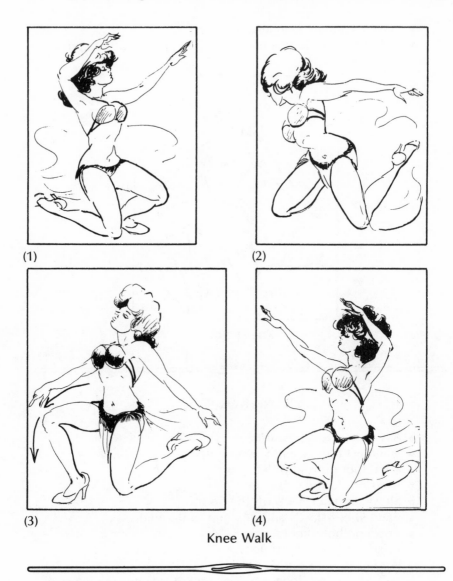

(1)

(2)

(3)

(4)

Knee Walk

Upper Torso Roll—Kneeling

- Assume correct posture.
- Stand with feet slightly apart, left foot in front of right foot.
- Descend to the floor slowly.
- Kneel on both knees.
- Bend over from the waist frontwards.
- Raise hands out in front.

- Bring head over to your right side; keep hands outstretched.
- Bring head around to the back.
- Bend your head backwards as far as you can.
- Swing head over to the left side.
- Return to bending position in front.
- This roll should be done as smoothly as possible.
- Repeat 4 times.

As you become better at this exercise, lower your upper torso until it almost reaches the floor. At the point where you actually touch the floor, use your hands to help push yourself along the floor.

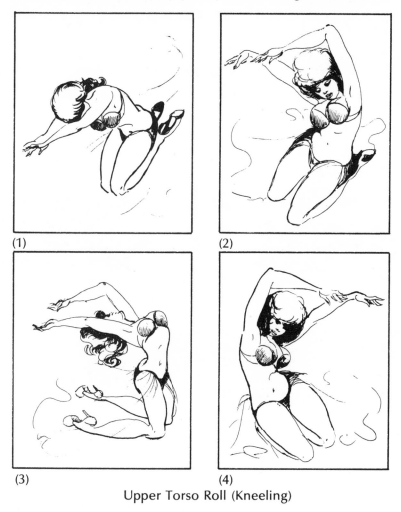

(1)   (2)

(3)   (4)

Upper Torso Roll (Kneeling)

Back Bend and Arch (Kneeling)

- Assume correct posture.
- Stand straight, feet slightly apart, left foot in front of right foot.
- Hands out to the sides.
- Slowly bend knees and descend to the floor.
- Kneel on both knees.
- Slowly lower your head backwards.
- Do not move your knees; grip the floor with them for balance.
- Lower head backwards; shoulders and torso follow in an arch.
- Lift head up, shoulders and torso back up to original position.
- Repeat 4 times.

Do not strain yourself. Each time you do this exercise, lower your torso a little more until it finally reaches the floor.

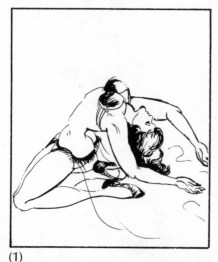
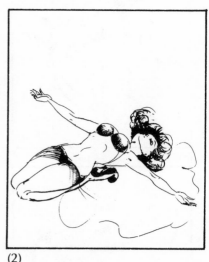

(1)   (2)

Back Bend and Arch (Kneeling)

Body Roll

- Assume correct posture.
- Start in a crouching position.
- Arch your back and suck in your stomach muscles.
- Tuck your head into your chest.
- Arms should be bent slightly in front of you.

- Bend your knees.
- Straighten your body slowly from the knees up.
- Raise your arms slowly up until they reach above your head.
- Release stomach muscles.
- Lower arms to sides.
- Repeat 5 times.

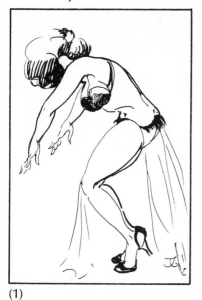

(1)

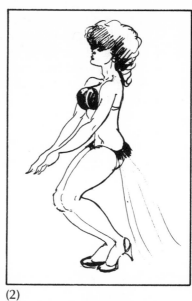

(2)

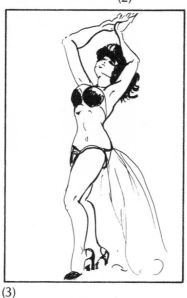

(3)

Body Roll

Pelvic Roll or Upper Torso Roll

- Assume correct posture.
- Stand with feet slightly apart.
- Arms out to the sides.
- Slide your pelvis out to the left.
- Push derriere out to the back.
- Bend forward from the waist down.
- Bring derriere around to the right.
- Tuck your derriere in under you.
- Push your pelvis out in front of you.
- Bend backwards, head back as far as you can.
- Slide over to the left.
- Return to starting position.
- Repeat 4 times.
- Do the same thing, starting the roll to the right.

You have the option of doing this exercise with a smooth flowing motion or emphasizing each position as you go along.

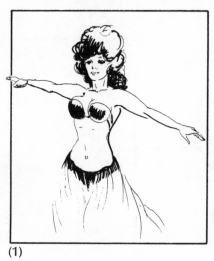

(1)

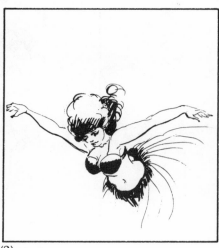

(2)

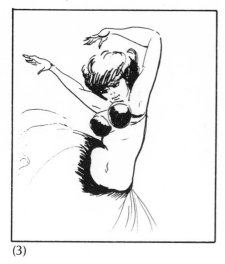

(3)

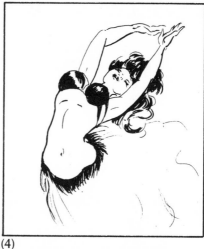

(4)

Pelvic Roll or Upper Torso Roll

Body Quiver

- Assume correct posture.
- Stand straight, feet slightly apart, left foot in front of right foot.
- Hands down at sides or bend elbows and bring hands to shoulders.
- Bend your left knee slightly.
- Straighten your right foot.
- Contract all your muscles in your right side and quiver the body.
- Increase the quiver until your whole body shakes.
- Continue for about 2 minutes.
- Straighten your left foot and do the same on this side.

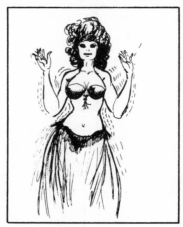

Body Quiver

Body Twist

- Assume correct posture.
- Stand straight, feet slightly apart, left foot in front of right foot.
- Hands down at sides or bend elbows and bring hands to shoulders.
- Slowly twist your derriere from side to side.
- Increase the movements until the lower part of the body is twisting. (This is the old Chubby Checker twist movement.)
- Continue for about 2 minutes.

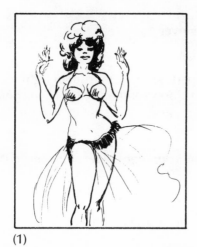

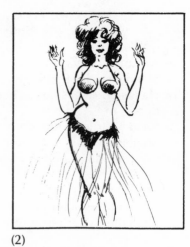

(1)   (2)
Body Twist

Serpent Crawl

- Assume horizontal position.
- Lie on your back; cross left leg on top of right leg.
- Hands out at sides.
- Dig right heel into floor; pull heels forward about 6 inches.
- Slowly dig derriere into the floor and pull it forward about 6 inches.
- Rib cage should be pulled up to form arch in your back.
- Shoulders remain on floor.
- Pull shoulders along 6 inches.
- Start crawl again.
- Dig heels into floor.
- Pull them forward 6 inches, then pull derriere 6 inches and then shoulders and head 6 inches.
- Repeat about 2 minutes until you have crawled across the floor.

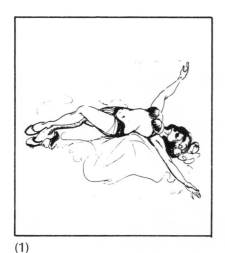
(1)

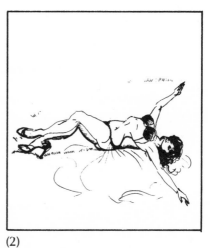
(2)

Serpent Crawl

Horizontal Knee Bends

- Assume horizontal position.
- Lie on your right side, hands outstretched above your head.
- Swing knees up and tuck them into the stomach.
- Hold for count of 4.
- Swing feet down and hold them straight.

- Repeat 4 times.
- Turn on left side and repeat exercise 4 times.

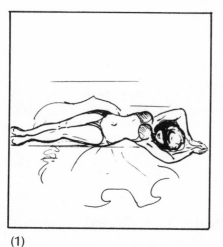
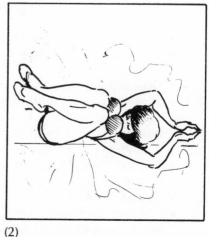

(1)   (2)

Horizontal Knee Bends

Horizontal Scissors Kick

- Assume horizontal position.
- Lie on your right side.
- Elevate your head.

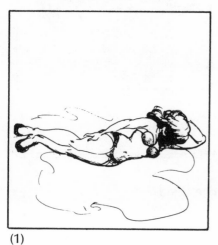
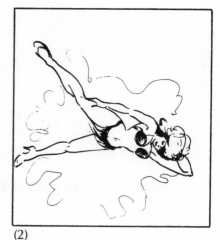

(1)   (2)

Horizontal Scissors Kick

- Bend your right arm and rest elbow on the floor.
- Rest your head on your hand.
- Leave left hand on top of your hip.
- Swing left foot up slowly in scissors kick.
- Hold for count of 3.
- Lower foot.
- Repeat 4 times.
- Turn on your left side and repeat same exercise raising your right foot 4 times.

Basic Circular Turn

- Assume correct posture.
- Stand straight, feet slightly apart, left foot in front of right foot.
- Step flat on the right foot.
- Tap the ball of the left foot as you turn towards the right.
- The ball of the left foot acts as a pivot and, therefore, should not move from place.
- Repeat about 8 times.
- Then step flat on the left foot and reverse the entire process.

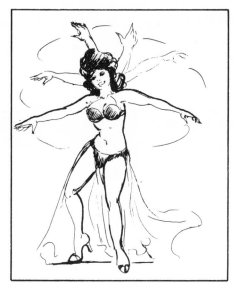

Basic Circular Turn

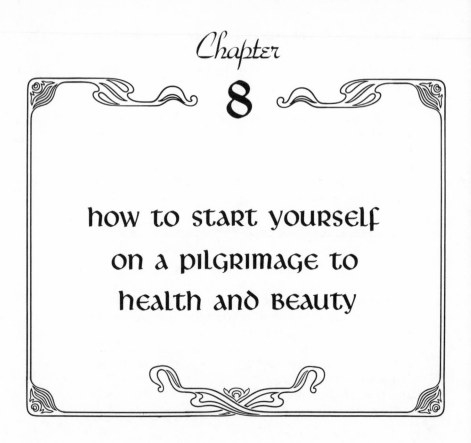

how to start yourself on a pilgrimage to health and beauty

How would you like to partake of an exotic journey without spending a cent? I thought that you might jump at an idea like that. Well, to "purchase" your ticket, motivation and self-determination are all you need to start on this exotic journey to an Arabian Nights fantasy and a lifetime of new and exciting dreams. Motivation and self-determination are your "American Express card." Your pilgrimage will be one of untold pleasures. Around every corner you will find exciting new ideas that will fill your life with a new zest, a new spark that no one will be able to extinguish once you have lit the flame.

But first, let us take time out for a "commercial" before you embark on your journey. I'd like to give you a little glimpse into your future so that you may see what marvelous treasures are in store for you. How would you like to be the social hostess supreme on your block and amongst your friends? I am going to show you how to be just that. Your ultimate goal will be giving an Arabian Nights gala for your friends and enemies. Yes, I said enemies, because there are going to be a lot of people at that party who are going to envy your new shape. Do not pay them any attention, just tell them how you did it. If they want to do it the Middle Eastern way, then fill their ears with your experiences and you will have made a follower out of them too. Then they will be on their way to a trim, healthy figure.

Later on I'm going to describe this Middle Eastern party to you. You are going to have a great deal of fun putting it together, and you will be so busy that you won't have time to nibble on all those fattening unhealthy goodies around the house. My advice to you would be to get rid of those goodies immediately because you do not need any tempting things around you, especially during the initial stages of your journey.

STARTING ON A JOURNEY

Okay, back to the business at hand. You are going to start yourself on a pilgrimage to health and exotic beauty. You are going to take on a whole new attitude and a whole new life. Your pilgrimage should take you about seven weeks. That's not too much time to take out of your life to fly on a magic carpet to a faraway land, is it?

A pilgrimage is a long journey, usually made to some sacred place as an act of devotion, such as the famous ones to Lourdes and Mecca. It can also be a journey that one undertakes in quest of something for a particular purpose, as to pay homage. You are going to embark on your pilgrimage in quest of a healthy and beautiful body. Your pilgrimage will be in quest of life, preserving it and living it to your fullest potential.

You can take your pilgrimage through the air, on water, or on land. I have chosen to take you down the Nile river, a waterway of ancient times that is still flowing along today full of its memories of yesterday.

Travel with me for a brief moment back in time, 4,000 years back into history to an ancient civilization that gave us paper, the 365-day calendar invented in response to the Nile river's annual flooding, ink, the waterwheel, and ultimately the greatest invention, I think— writing. Where would we be without it? My goodness, this book wouldn't be possible! Writing was the invention of the people of Mesopotamia and Egypt. Let us take a ride down the Nile of ancient times, the longest river in the world. Yes, the Nile, which even today has the largest of all engineering projects—the two-mile-long Aswan dam which will double Egypt's power of production. The Nile, full of waterlilies and lotus. You are the queen of all you survey, you are waited on hand and foot by your handmaidens, stuffing you full of grapes, nuts, and other healthy foods. They didn't have popcorn then, thank goodness; you ate of the fruits of the land and were well nourished. Your skin was bathed with milk and honey. You didn't have to worry about your rent bill and the expenses. You didn't have to worry about the amount of red dye # 2 in your food. All you ever thought about was how beautiful you were going to make yourself.

Now, keep floating down that ancient river with its peaceful waters lapping against the sides of your royal barge. But now, I would like you to transfer your body to your bathtub; your mind should still be in the Middle East because I would like you to have an experience I am sure you have never had before. You are going to explore your body in a way you have never done before.

AN EXPERIENCE IN YOUR BATH

Fill your bathtub with the most exotic oils or gelée you have. I personally use Badedas (Vita Bath Gelée)—it is the most refreshing product I have ever used in my bath. If you want to be more exotic you could use some of the Middle Eastern aromas, such as jasmine, chypre, secret of the desert, heliotrope, or musk, that are found in specialty shops. Now, you are going to immerse your entire body in this exotic body of water that is all yours. Nobody is there to interrupt your privacy. Just lie there and let your pores cleanse themselves and soak up the magnificent moisture and aroma.

There are very few people who take this part of their life seriously or have stopped to give it a second thought. When was the last time that you really thought about the kind of bath you were going to take? I would like to give you the opportunity on this pilgrimage to stop awhile and give your body an experience—an absolution that you will keep repeating for a long, long time. This will be something that you will cherish all your life. I promise you that from this day forward you will look forward to your bath with a new sense of purpose. It will become much more than an act of washing away a few specks of dirt.

WHAT WATER DOES FOR YOU

Water soothes the body. You take a shower, you feel better; you wash your face, you feel better; you wash your hair, you feel better, and so forth. Water running on your body produces a sort of kneading motion that tones your skin. It helps you to feel tingly and refreshed all over. Thales of Miletus (600 B.C.) said that water was the source of all things. I would like to attach as much importance as he did to water and make it be a source of energy for your body.

In the Bible, Jesus used water as a symbol in the baptism ceremony. He washed his disciples' feet with water. Water was used in a deep and significant form of purification. The Moslems wash their hands and feet before entering the mosque to pray. Even before we start our life's journey on earth we are surrounded by water in our mother's womb, and water flows through our bodies until the day we die. The longest anyone has ever lived without water was ten days. Without water I daresay there would be no life. Water is a source for our food and it serves as a highway for travel.

We drink water, we bathe in it, it irrigates our deserts, and it runs our industrial plants. It is the life blood of our industry—we depend on it to help cool the steel that makes our automobiles, it washes impurities from pulp in paper mills, and it supplies the warmth that radiates from some of our heating systems, and so it goes. It surrounds our land, falls down from the sky, and gushes out of our land. It can be a liquid, a gas, or it can even be turned into a solid. The first civilizations sprung up around water—the Nile of Egypt, the Indus of Northern India, the Tigris-Euphrates of Mesopotamia (modern Iraq), and the Yellow River or Hwang Ho of China, for example. Think of the over 370 million Hindus who make pilgrimages to the holy Ganges River to wash in its waters at least once during their lives.

You too are going to make water work for you. After you have soaked yourself for awhile you are going to start your water exercises. The benefit of doing these exercises in the water is that the water acts as a counterforce against which you do your exercise, thus giving your muscles more resistance and hence a better workout.

Your body must welcome these exercises, not resist them. The only resistance you want with the water exercises is that which you get through the water itself.

Here I must tell you the story of my dear friend Jackie P. She had a rather large potbelly which she just could not get rid of no matter how little food she ate. Now, you must believe me when I tell you that she spends at least one hour in the bathroom taking a bath. This was her way of relaxing after a hard day's work.

Well, one day I had a brainstorm. I was working on the water exercises for my book and I asked her if she would help me test them out. Seeing a chance to have a new expereince in the bathtub, she gladly helped me. After only one week of these exercises she lost 5 pounds. Evidently, she enjoyed them so much that she did them diligently and they really helped her.

Guess where she lost the 5 pounds? Her potbelly disappeared! If Jackie P. can do it, so can you. Exercise was not her thing in life. The fact is that she was having so much fun doing them that she forgot that she was exercising.

Since all my exercises are accompanied by music I would like to suggest a few records for these exercises. My favorite Middle Eastern records for these exercises are the following:

1. *Impressions of the Middle East*—Herbie Mann—Atlantic.
2. *Babylon Mood*—Munir Bechir and his Quartet—Parlophone—Voix De l'Orient

Herbie Mann handles his impressions of the Middle East with a hint of jazz running through the exotic tunes. If you like Herbie Mann you'll love this record; if you dig jazz, you'll love this record. This record will serve as a great introduction to the sounds of the Middle East because Herbie Mann has handled it with a delicacy that will weave a spell over your senses.

Babylon Mood has an extremely lovely side 1. The music is slow and beautiful and is perfect for lulling your mind while the water of your bath laps over your body as you do your exercises. I like the idea of having the cassette tape going right near the bathtub, but be sure that it is battery operated to avoid electrical mishaps. You too should react to this musical interlude with your bath in a very pleasant manner. Bring the music close to your bathtub so that it can soothe you while you are exercising your cares and excess pounds away.

These exercises are for the standard-size bathtub. If you're one of the lucky ones who has an oversized tub, adjust your exercises accordingly. If you have a heart-shaped bathtub you're going to have a lot of extra adjustments to make. Watch out for the point of the heart! You are going to have to do your exercises sort of sideways in the bathtub.

Here are a few safety suggestions so that you will make your water exercises a safe and pleasant experience:

1. Don't fill your bathtub with too much water. I find that a good amount is about one inch more than half full so that you will have enough water in the bathtub to offer resistance but not enough to splatter the bathroom floor or to cover your head.
2. Keep your head above the water at all times. You may feel more comfortable if you rest it on the side of the tub and sort of grip the edge of the bathtub with your neck for some of the

exercises. If that's not comfortable hold your head straight up out of the water.

3. Your feet should always be towards the faucet to prevent you from bumping your head on it.
4. Your hands and elbows should be used to help you keep your balance at all times.
5. Keep such items as soaps and back scratchers away from the bathtub. You don't want objects falling into the bathtub while you're doing your exercises. They may cause you to slip and may injure your body.
6. Keep electrical appliances away from the water to avoid dangerous accidents. You could use an electrically run tape recorder in a room nearby and just have the music float into the bathroom until you are doing your exercises.
7. When you slide back and forth be careful not to move backwards too quickly, as you could bump your head on the side of the bathtub.

If you are trying to lose weight, you should do all the following exercises at least twice a week, preferably every day. They should take about 15 minutes. For the days in-between, cut down the exercise time to 10 minutes.

If you are trying to maintain your weight, 10 minutes each day of the water exercises should be enough.

Now get ready for an exciting trip into ecstasyland.

Water Exercise # 1

- Lie flat on your back in the bathtub, with head just above water.
- Head resting on the back edge of the bathtub.
- Back against the wall of bathtub.
- Close your eyes and think pleasant thoughts.
- Hands flat on the floor of the bathtub, palms up.
- Relax completely for a slow count of 25.

Water Exercise # 2

- Lie flat on your back in the bathtub, with head just above water.
- Head resting on the back edge of the bathtub.

- Back against the wall of bathtub.
- Feet 6" up the faucet side of the tub.
- Feet flat on the side of the bathtub.
- Knees bent and together.
- Hands flat on floor of bathtub.
- Straighten knees, push head up.
- Bend knees, pull buttocks down towards heels.
- Repeat this bending and sliding motion 5 times.

Water Exercise # 3

- Lie flat on your back in the bathtub, with head just above water.
- Head straight up.
- Assume a semi-sitting position, shoulders out of water.
- Back against wall of bathtub.
- Hands on hips.
- Bend knees, straighten knees.
- Repeat this bending motion 5 times.

Water Exercise # 4

- Lie flat on your back in the bathtub, with head just above water.
- Head straight up.
- Assume a semi-sitting position.
- Back against wall of bathtub.
- Rest heels about 6" up on the faucet side of the bathtub.
- Feet flat on the side of the bathtub.
- Hands on hips.
- Push hips to the right side until buttocks touch side of the bathtub.
- Hold for count of 2.
- Push hips to the left side until buttocks touch side of the bathtub.
- Hold for count of 2.
- Repeat 5 times on each side.

Water Exercise # 5

- Lie flat on back in the bathtub, with head just above water.
- Head barely touching edge of bathtub.
- Elbows on bottom of bathtub.
- Hands holding hips.
- Knees bent.
- Bottom of feet on floor of bathtub.
- Slide buttocks down until they nearly touch the heels.
- Hands slide up your sides.
- Repeat 5 times.

Water Exercise # 6

- Lie flat on back in the bathtub, with head just above water.
- Head touching edge of bathtub.
- Back against wall of bathtub, press shoulders against back of bathtub.
- Buttocks in palms of hands.
- Legs straight out.
- Bottom of feet on side of bathtub.
- Bend right foot until leg touches your chest—knee touching face.
- Hold for count of 2.
- Straighten legs.
- Same thing on left side.
- Alternate feet.
- Repeat 5 times on each side.

Water Exercise # 7

- Lie flat on back in bathtub, with head just above water.
- Head touching edge of bathtub, back against back wall of bathtub.
- Hands flat on floor of bathtub.
- Heels against floor of bathtub.
- Bottom of feet on side of bathtub.

- Pull feet straight up out of water without bending knees.
- Hold for count of 2.
- Lower feet slowly.
- Repeat 5 times.

Water Exercise # 8

- Same exercise as above, but alternate feet and do one foot at a time in a sort of scissors motion.

Water Exercise # 9

- Lie flat on back in bathtub, with head just above water.
- Bottom of feet on side of bathtub.
- Buttocks in hands.
- Neck resting on side of bathtub.
- Knees bent, rest them on side of bathtub.
- Legs spread apart.
- Heels on floor of bathtub.
- Slide buttocks down until they almost touch the heels.
- Slide buttocks back up to starting position.
- Repeat 5 times.

Water Exercise # 10

- Lie flat on back in bathtub, with head just above water.
- Back against wall of bathtub, press shoulders against back of bathtub.
- Buttocks in hands.
- Bottom of feet on floor of bathtub.
- Knees bent.
- Legs spread open, knees touching sides of bathtub.
- Bring knees together, then open knees again.
- Repeat opening and closing motions 5 times.

Water Exercise # 11

- Assume seated position, back straight up against edge of bathtub.
- Bottom of feet flat on side of bathtub.
- Legs straight and together.
- Rest hands on floor of bathtub.
- Bend right knee and pull it up as far as possible to your chest with both hands, fingers interlocked.
- Hold for count of 2.
- Repeat bending motion 5 times.
- Same thing on left side.

Water Exercise # 12

- This is similar to Exercise # 4, but should be done a little faster without holding positions.
- Assume seated position.
- Head and shoulders straight, press firmly against side of bathtub.
- Bottom of feet flat on edge of bathtub.
- Hold buttocks in hands.
- Swing buttocks around to the right until they touch the side of the bathtub.
- Slide buttocks back until they are flat on floor of bathtub.
- Swing buttocks around to the left until they touch left side of tub.
- Right, left, right, left.
- Repeat 5 times.

Water Exercise # 13

- Assume seated position.
- Head up, back away from edge of bathtub.
- Hands on knees.
- Feet stretched straight out.
- Bottom of feet on faucet side of bathtub.
- Grab hold of the faucet handles with both hands.

- Pull yourself up in a sliding motion towards faucets.
- Slide buttocks towards heels of feet.
- Push yourself back to starting position.
- Slide buttocks down to heels again.
- Repeat 5 times.

Water Exercise # 14

- Lie flat on stomach, with head just above water.
- Head up.
- Knees bent.
- Feet up out of the water.
- Inside of elbows on bottom of bathtub.
- Hands flat on floor of bathtub.
- Pull yourself up and forward until the chin touches the side of the bathtub.
- Push yourself back.
- Up and back.
- Repeat 5 times.

Water Exercise # 15

- Lie flat on stomach, with head just above water.
- Arms folded in front of you.
- Elbows on bottom of bathtub.
- Face down.
- Knees bent.
- Toes on wall on faucet side of bathtub.
- Pull your knees up towards chest.
- Assume a sort of praying position.
- Slide yourself down until knees touch edge of bathtub at bottom of bathtub.
- Slide up, buttocks in air, praying position, straighten out and slide back.
- Repeat 5 times.

Water Exercise # 16

- Lie on left side, with head just above water.
- Left elbow bent, hand flat on floor of bathtub.
- Knees bent until touching left side of bathtub.
- Grab your right ankle with right hand and pull your right knee up to your chest.
- Hold for count of 5.
- Return to starting position.
- Repeat 5 times.
- Lie on right side.
- Grab your left ankle.
- Pull up and back.
- Repeat 5 times.

Water Exercise # 17

- Lie on left side, with head just above water.
- Left elbow bent, hand flat on floor of bathtub.
- Knees bent until touching left side of bathtub.
- Grab the under side of your right foot.
- Straighten leg up out of the water.
- Hold for count of 5.
- Return leg to starting position.
- Repeat 5 times.
- Lie on right side, grab left foot, and repeat exercise on this side.

Water Exercise # 18

- Lie flat on back, with head just above water.
- Knees bent up out of water.
- Heels flat on floor of tub.
- Hands flat on floor of bathtub.
- Head on side of bathtub.
- Shoulders touching side of bathtub.
- Bring your rib cage up out of water as far as you can, arch your back, shoulders come away from edge of bathtub.

- Hold for count of 10.
- Lower rib cage.
- Return to starting position.
- Repeat 5 times.

Water Exercise # 19

- Lie flat on back, with head just above water.
- Shoulders touching side of bathtub.
- Relax, hands at sides.
- Bend knees and rest them on sides of bathtub.
- Pull stomach in, breathe out.
- Hold for count of 2.
- Push stomach out, breathe in.
- Hold for count of 2.
- Repeat 5 times.
- Relax.

Water Exercise # 20

- Turn tap on with warm water.
- Lie flat on back, with head just above water.
- Buttocks in palms of hands.
- Place your left foot close to the faucet and let water beat down between your toes.
- Hold for count of 10.
- Make tap water cold.
- Let cold tap water run through your toes.
- Hold for count of 5.
- Repeat with right foot.
- Repeat 5 times.

Water Exercise # 21

- Assume seated position.
- Back straight up out of water.
- Turn on tap, make water warm.

- Hold fingers under water and let water beat down on them.
- Hold for count of 10.
- Make tap water cold.
- Let cold water run through your fingers.
- Hold for count of 5.

BRUSH STIMULATION

When you are through with these water exercises, get under the shower and let the water beat down on your body so that it can massage every pore in your skin and thus stimulate your blood circulation. Make the water as hot as you can bear it, then gradually make it cooler until it's cold and makes your body start to tingle. You will experience an utter tranquility and exhilaration beyond words. Help this action along by taking a body brush and massaging every inch of your body except your breasts. This is fantastic for your blood circulation. You should start seeing significant results in the way your body feels, the way your soul feels and the way your mind feels. To keep your skin smooth, apply a mild oil to every inch of your body. The massaging effect will further enhance your skin tone. Even the lowliest lady in Egypt used to bathe herself in oil because of the dryness of the Egyptian climate. The more highly placed ladies lavished themselves with frankincense and myrrh. Yes, frankincense and myrrh. This goes back to Biblical days. In Exodus, God told Moses to take unto him sweet spices with pure frankincense, and throughout the Bible the sweet smells of these two oils are mentioned over and over.

Now, we slowly leave that serene environment of a water-soaked existence and slowly come back to this century, but don't leave that part of the world yet. Now picture yourself in a casbah somewhere in the Middle East, with the muezzin chanting his call to prayer—one of the most moving sounds I have ever heard in my life. Imagine that he is calling to you, not to pray, although it might indeed help you to gain some faith, but to wake up to the realization that you are going to become a new person. He is calling to you to change your way of life, calling you to a life of health and beauty, calling to you to abstain from unhealthy substances, and he is calling you to exercise your whole body and keep it fit.

GETTING EVERYBODY INVOLVED

Come home now, to your home town, and get started on your local journey. Your ticket took you to a faraway land and now you are back to your immediate goal. Remember that your ultimate goal is to be more than just the hostess at your Arabian Nights party—you are going to be the star with a new body. Wait until your friends see you in your new Oriental dance costume; they are going to flip over you. Chances are they won't recognize you. That should be fun. If you are married and have a husband who could handle this kind of surprise, keep the whole affair a secret from him until that magical day. If you feel he could not, then let him in on the "secret" beforehand. You don't want him huffing and puffing in a corner when you spring the surprise on your friends and on him.

Of course you are going to involve him in your new-found knowledge on the health and exercise aspect of the program. As I said before, men can get involved in this routine too. (Don't let him carry it too far, though. We don't want him parading around in an Oriental dance costume!) These exercises and eating patterns are good for the teenagers in the family also. Get everybody involved.

You have your ticket to begin your pilgrimage now. The next thing you are going to do is to add to your ticket the places you expect to go. Get a picture of an Oriental dancer that has all the right bulges in the right places. You can get this in one of many ways—either buy a Middle Eastern album with one of those gorgeous creatures on the album cover, get a picture from a friend who is a dancer, get a picture from your nearest Oriental dance studio, have a friend sketch a picture of you (the svelte version) in an Oriental dance costume, or just look at some of the pictures in my book (I had to get in a plug for myself there!) and copy one of them. Tack this picture up on the front of your refrigerator and on the door of any closet behind which hides your favorite cookie jar or some other such unhealthy, fattening product. This will be part of your ticket to remind you of where you have to go with your weight. When you go to that refrigerator door, just look at that picture and think of that great party you're going to star in, and don't even open the door. Go away and start sewing that dress you've been meaning to start, or better yet, start making your Oriental dance costume for the big event at your house. If you get past the refrigerator door, then make sure that you have some raw vegetables sliced in appetizing tidbits to come out with in your little hands. These vegetables are extremely healthy for you and should satisfy your craving. Don't overdo it, though. It would be a good idea to keep them in front of the shelf and place the more fattening things in the back, out of reach.

PUTTING FASTENERS ON YOUR COSTUME

You can delay putting on the hooks and other fasteners on your costume until you achieve your desired measurement, or if you do put them on, put on a few spare rows. As a matter of course I put on two rows of hooks on all my costumes because my weight fluctuates a little too. That second row of hooks on all my costumes has also served as a face-saving device on the few occasions that my bra decided that it had enough and went "snap." Yes, that has happened to me! Fortunately for me it wasn't too embarassing a situation because the hooks just settled into the second set of eyes. You see, perspiration weakens the threads on the hooks and eyes, and if you do not check your costume regularly for worn thread, they can sometimes break at a very inopportune moment.

After you have taken off the pounds you desire, your fluctuation in weight should never be too great—no more than four or five pounds one way or the other. If your weight goes up and down more than that, you are cheating and eating or dieting too much. The idea is to keep a fairly constant weight, not one that goes up and down like the Dow-Jones averages.

The next step on your ticket should be one of informing yourself of the culture and history of the Middle East and its surrounding areas. I have provided you with a little background, but that is by far not enough. You will get into the swing of things if you really feel the mood of that part of the world. You have to feel the music, you have to feel the people, you have to feel the culture, you have to feel the history, and I would really like you to get very involved with the food of the area. I want you to experience the music in such a way that whenever you hear it you will want to get up and dance. I want you to exercise your body, and I want you to exercise your mind.

Start stocking your kitchen cabinets with things Middle Eastern, Greek, and Turkish. Start purchasing some more Middle Eastern records. Visit your local Middle Eastern, Greek, or Turkish restaurant. The great thing about my plan is that you can go out and enjoy a good meal in a restaurant without becoming guilt-ridden about it. The only word of caution I would have for you is that you should watch the portions you eat and of course be sure that you eat a balanced meal. Remember, it is not necessary for you to starve yourself to death when you try to lose weight the Oriental dancer's way. Start taking in the performances of Oriental dancers and pay particular attention to how supple they are. You too can achieve their suppleness.

You are going to give yourself seven weeks to achieve your desired goal, and promise me that you are going to follow my instructions religiously. I am counting on you. Don't let me down. Don't let yourself down.

Your doctor can tell you what your desired weight should be according to your age and build, and he can guide you through the difficult times. Check the chart included here to give you a general idea of what your weight should be.

Desirable Weights for Men and Women Age 25 and Over

Adapted from the Metropolitan Life Insurance Co., New York.
New weight standards for men and women.
Statistical Bulletin 40:3.

Men

Height		Small Frame	Medium Frame	Large Frame
Feet	Inches			
5	2	112-120	118-129	126-141
5	3	115-123	121-133	129-144
5	4	118-126	124-136	132-148
5	5	121-129	127-139	135-152
5	6	124-133	130-143	138-156
5	7	128-137	134-147	142-161
5	8	132-141	138-152	147-166
5	9	136-145	142-156	151-170
5	10	140-150	146-160	155-174
5	11	144-154	150-165	159-179
6	0	148-158	154-170	164-184
6	1	152-162	158-175	168-189
6	2	156-167	162-180	173-194
6	3	160-171	167-185	178-199
6	4	164-175	172-190	182-204

Women

Height		Small Frame	Medium Frame	Large Frame
Feet	Inches			
4	10	92-98	96-107	104-119
4	11	94-101	98-110	106-122
5	0	96-104	101-113	109-125
5	1	99-107	104-116	112-128
5	2	102-110	107-119	115-131
5	3	105-113	110-122	118-134
5	4	108-116	113-126	121-138
5	5	111-119	116-130	125-142
5	6	114-123	120-135	129-146
5	7	118-127	124-139	133-150
5	8	122-131	128-143	137-154
5	9	126-135	132-147	141-158
5	10	130-140	136-151	145-163
5	11	134-144	140-155	149-168
6	0	138-148	144-159	153-173

During the first few weeks of your pilgrimage, try to lose about three pounds per week. You want to go slowly at first because the pounds you take off are going to stay off. During the last three weeks try for a goal of four pounds per week. If you need to lose more than 25 pounds let your pilgrimage take you a little longer; there should be no hurry. You and your doctor can work out a timetable of weight loss. Since each person is different this difference should be taken into consideration at all times. Remember that what's good for the goose may not be good for the gander. I would like you to find a comfortable regimen to follow. I do not want you sliding back into your old ways. If it means that you take a little longer on your journey that's fine.

Early in this pilgrimage you have to decide whether you are going to embark on a *reducing* eating pattern or a *maintaining* eating pattern. You will have to decide whether you have to shed pounds or just keep the pounds you have in tip-top shape.

On a reducing eating pattern you will increase your exercises so that they burn up more calories than you consume. Your scale is going to be a very useful partner on this venture. After you get the hang of balancing food intake and exercise, you won't need to use the scale—you will know exactly what to do.

In order to lose three pounds the first week you'll have to lose approximately half a pound each day. If you don't lose any pounds the first day, increase your exercises by five minutes the next day, keeping your food intake constant. The key word here is *balance*. You must achieve a balance between your food intake and energy release.

On a maintaining eating pattern the line is even finer, and a more sophisticated regulating pattern is necessary. You will exercise moderately and eat moderately.

If you have a craving for some particular food item, your body probably needs the nutrient derived from that product. You run into difficulty when this craving is no longer the real craving of the body but is a craving of the mind. You see, your mind does not really need the food—your mind has no teeth to chew "body" food—but it needs nourishment, so sometimes your mind gets confused as to what kind of nourishment it should have. Instead of feeding itself with the correct food—stimulating information to exercise its cells—your mind convinces you that you need some chocolates, a slice of pizza, or a thick ice cream sundae. You do not need any of these. Fight these cravings with great determination.

Remember that the hypothalamus governs many processes that do not wait for conscious decisions, such as sleeping and waking, appetite, heart action, sex, digestion, and thirst. In case you have forgotten, the hypothalamus is housed in the base of the brain. There are two cell groups here, one initiates the urge to eat and the other counteracts the urge. In some people this latter group doesn't work properly, and that's when you continue eating without any control. It maintains water balance by a process which regulates the kidneys and stimulates the nerves at the back of the throat. It is possible to feel no thirst at all if your throat is kept moist.

It is very important to keep the water balance in the body. You lose water from the body in many different ways. It is exhaled in your breath, through perspiration, and by direct excretion. In order to survive you must balance the loss by drinking approximately five to six pints of water every day. The most vital function that water performs in the body is in the kidneys, where it purges wastes from the bloodstream. About 2,000 quarts of blood are "washed" each day. If one kidney fails, the other one can do its job; however, if both fail then you are in a lot of trouble—you can't live for more than three weeks with uncleaned blood.

Cure yourself of your craving for sweets. They are chock full of sugar and you must stay away from that product. If you feel that you cannot overcome this urge, keep a jar of honey handy and take a level teaspoon whenever you must have something sweet. Honey is a natural product and thus helps to soothe your stomach. A teaspoon taken before bedtime can relax you and calm your nerves. It helps to preserve the vitamins in your system. Moreover, honey contains ten of the amino acids considered essential to people. It also helps to improve your health by acting as a regulatory agent. It acts as a balance in your bodily functions—it helps to fight diarrhea and also acts as a gentle laxative. It is a great substitute for sugar, but like anything else, do not overdo eating honey either.

What you feed into your body is very important. You cannot achieve respect for your body by doing exercises alone. On your pilgrimage you are going to eat foods with a Middle Eastern flavor to them, but by no means are you going to exclude other foods. I have found that the Middle Eastern, Turkish, and Greek kitchen provides us with an abundant amount of nutrients. Take another look at some of the products that one associates with these cultures: olives, dates, almonds, figs, lamb, wheat, feta cheese (made with goat's milk) peaches, yogurt, and others. Man's original diet consisted of fruit, nuts, grains, and vegetables. I think that it is about time that we returned to some of the original things in life. It seems that every other week someone comes out with some "new" food substance that is supposed to end all your weight and health problems. Most of them are just fads that gain your interest for a short period of time and then disappear into oblivion. I am asking you to get back to the basics of the earth—fruits, nuts, grains, and vegetables.

Nutrition is as old as the Bible. Throughout the Bible we are warned against improper eating. (If this concept of nutrition or eating properly has been around for so long, maybe there is some validity to it.) The Bible even gives you a case history to prove that eating meat is not always good for you. Daniel did an experiment for Melzar. Daniel forbade his followers to eat any of the king's meat for ten days, and at the end of ten days their countenances appeared fairer and fatter in flesh than all the children that did eat the portion of the king's meat. This case history can be found in Chapter 1 of the Book of Daniel.

I am by no means a vegetarian, but I don't think that you should eat too much meat. In the Middle East they stretch their meats with vegetables through necessity, because meat is so expensive; but inevitably this process is healthier.

Angelina M. had converted to a religion that does not permit her to eat meat. She found the transition to total abstinence extremely difficult, as a woman in her late 50's who was trying to reduce her meat intake drastically after a lifetime of gorging herself with thick steaks. We were talking about this problem one day, and I suggested that she kill two birds with one stone and go the Middle Eastern way. I suggested that she stretch her meat dishes by adding lots of vegetables to them. Angelina tried this, and she hasn't stopped talking about how this helped her to finally maintain a meat-free eating pattern and to lose her extra pounds. I was so happy that I could help her, even though I do not advocate the total rejection of meat.

God tells us that we are the temple of God and we should be destroyed if we defile that temple. That's what your pilgrimage is all about. You are taking it to cleanse your souls and your bodies. You also want to improve your mind, and if your body is not healthy, your mind cannot function the way it should.

Before the flood God let the people eat the ox, the sheep, and the goat, but no other animals. He also said that people could eat all things in the sea that have fins and scales, but everything else would be unclean and therefore unfit to eat. They could also eat all clean birds. After the flood he warned against eating meats because the animals were considered contaminated. That's why some religions advocate a meatless eating pattern. God also warns us against unclean fresh foods, intoxicating drinks, and tobacco and narcotics.

A great deal of the fish in the Middle East is just fantastic. In Chapter 11 you will find some delicious recipes for your eating pleasure.

If you eat the right foods you will be on your way to improving your body tone, and within seven weeks you will float off on your royal barge with exhilarating, stimulating, invigorating, electrifying, and glowing skin that is lit from within.

Water always fascinated me because of its many-faceted purposes—you can bathe in it, wash clothes with it, drink it, it serves as the home for a million different species of fish, it gives us power, and it waters our earth. It is the only substance without which we cannot live.

The earth is also bountiful with foods. Eat of them in a sensible way and you will prosper for a long time.

FOODS LOW IN CALORIES

Although we are not counting calories with this eating plan, it would be useful to keep in mind which foods are low in calories. It doesn't make too much sense to eat excessively rich foods that are chock full of calories and then have to spend half your life exercising in order to burn up the added energy. On the other hand, you do not have to exclude rich foods completely. Listed here are some low-calorie foods that you should plan to make more use of in your eating pattern.

Dairy Products
cottage cheese
whole milk
plain yogurt
camembert cheese
Edam cheese
buttermilk
non-fat reconstituted skim milk

Fruits
apples
apricots, fresh or dried
bananas
blueberries
cantaloupes
currants
figs
raw cherries
grapefruit
grapes
honeydew melon
lemons
limes
oranges
peaches
pears
prunes, dried
raspberries
strawberries
tangerines
watermelon
fruit cocktail, canned
raisins

Fruit Products
apple juice, frozen or canned
applesauce, frozen or canned

grapefruit juice
orange juice, fresh
tomato juice, canned

Grain Products
Oatmeal, cooked

Baked and Cooked Products
pumpkin pie
spaghetti, cooked

Meat and Meat Products
chili con carne
corn beef hash, canned
liver, beef

Fish and Seafoods
bluefish, baked
clams, raw
flounder, raw
haddock, cooked
lobster, canned
oysters, raw
scallops, broiled
shrimp, canned
tuna, canned

Eggs and Poultry
eggs, whole, raw
chicken, roasted

Vegetables
asparagus, cooked
beans, lima, cooked
beet greens
broccoli, cooked
Brussels sprouts
cabbage

carrots, raw
cauliflower
celery, raw
corn
cucumber
endive
escarole
lettuce, headed
mushrooms, raw
onions, mature, cooked
parsley
peas, green, cooked
pepper, sweet, green
potatoes, white, boiled

radishes
spinach, cooked, raw
string beans
tomatoes, raw
turnip greens
watercress

Miscellaneous

almonds
coffee, black
tea

Beverages (alcoholic)

White wine, claret or chablis

These are some of the foods that you should stock for your pilgrimage. After all, you will need food for your seven-week voyage.

Now, just let me briefly sum up some of the main points of this chapter.

1. "Purchase" your ticket to a healthy and happy body with motivation and self-determination.
2. Take a look into the future.
3. Travel down the Nile river to the roots of where it all began.
4. Begin to get the feeling of the Middle East, Greece, and Turkey in your blood.
5. Familiarize yourself with your goals and stick to them.
6. Discover a whole new world in your bathtub—water exercises will help you stay healthy and beautiful.
7. Start stocking your kitchen cabinets with things Middle Eastern.
8. Visit your local Middle Eastern, Greek, and Turkish restaurants.
9. Keep a lookout for performances of Oriental dancers.
10. Follow some of the eating hints to help you keep trim.
11. Plan healthy low-calorie foods for your eating pleasure.

Now you are well on your way to a life of health and beauty. Plan to take many a pleasurable, rewarding pilgrimage.

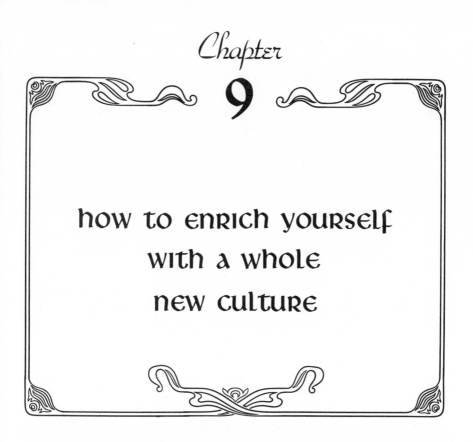

Chapter

9

how to enrich yourself with a whole new culture

One of my first introductions to the importance of the delicacy we call yogurt was on the streets of Istanbul, Turkey. At the time I was living there with my husband and young daughter. One day I was walking down the street and heard a man's shrieking voice calling out some mumbled jargon. I couldn't imagine what he was saying until finally, as he came closer, I made out the word "yoğurtçu" (pronounced yo-urt-ju). Up came this man with a little box, ringing his bell to draw the attention of passersby. Out came a little cup of white stuff. I had eaten yogurt at home and I was never a fancier of the stuff, but since the man was obviously making his living selling this product, it seemed to me that it must be something very special indeed. Lo and behold, it wasn't bad at all. Then and there I became a yogurt fan.

While we were in Turkey, my daughter also became "hooked" on yogurt. I remember her leaning out of the living room window and calling out to the yogurt man, "yoğurtçu." This meant "yogurt man" in Turkish. One could compare him to the ice cream man here in the United States. The children in Turkey look forward to the yogurt man as much as the children here in the United States look forward to the ice cream man. As one deeply aware of nutrition, I must say that yogurt is far healthier than the sugar-filled ice cream that we push on the streets of every town during the summer months. Of course adding all that sugar to the ice cream turns me off completely, and to add insult to injury, American children are encouraged to have hot sweet chocolate, sprinkles, and other poor nutrients smothered over the already sugary ice cream.

THE STORY OF A MIRACULOUS FOOD

Through my research I found that the use of yogurt originated with the Persian nomads. In the heat of that area, yogurt was much easier to keep on their travels than plain milk. Evidently it was a very integral part of their eating pattern.

It is said that yogurt was brought to this country by some Turks in 1784. The Greeks have also had a long association with this product.

Elie Metchnikoff, a Russian Nobel Prize winner, did some experiments at the Pasteur Institute in France in the 1900s. He believed that the yogurt bacteria worked in the stomach to prevent poisonous bacteria from growing there. He was also experimenting with the relationship of yogurt to longevity. He found that the Bulgarians ate a great deal of yogurt, and that many of them lived to be extremely old. This led Metchnikoff to link yogurt intake with longevity.

From Metchnikoff's experiments in 1919, a Spaniard named Isaac Carasso started manufacturing yogurt in Barcelona, Spain. This business spread to France and finally in 1942 to the United States. Today the market is flooded with many brand names. Dannon Yogurt remains my favorite because it doesn't use any artificial additives, and this was their policy even before it became the popular fashion.

If you have ever seen some of the commercials for Dannon Yogurt you will see an added reason why it has gained more prestige with me. The commercial with the men and women 90-140 years old from the Republic of Abkhazia in the Soviet Union is my favorite. I just adore them, and I figure if yogurt is such a big staple in their eating pattern then it's good enough for me. As the Dannon Yogurt people say about their commercials, "It is not only yogurt that is being sold through these commercials, but also the joyful experience of eating yogurt."

In Turkey, Greece, Lebanon and many other Middle Eastern countries, you put yogurt on *everything*—eggs, rice, spinach and meats, for example. The only "no-no" for Middle Easterners is fish—never on fish, folks. As I mentioned before, it is sold in the streets in its natural state; however, by now I'm sure they too are using the flavored versions that are so popular here in the United States.

The word "yogurt" is a Turkish word, *yoḡurt* (the g is silent). In Armenia the same substance is called *madzoon* (mazoun or mazun). In Persia it is known as *most*. Elsewhere in the Middle East it is called *laban*. It is and has been one of the principal foods of this section of the world for a long, long time dating back to Biblical times. Yogurt is mentioned in the Bible as laban. It probably became popular in that part of the world because refrigeration was not that good, and yogurt does not sour as easily as milk.

BENEFITS OF A MIRACULOUS FOOD

Yogurt should not be considered a cure-all for everything, but its nutritional benefits have all been well documented. Some nutritionists claim that it helps to immunize against bacteria. Someone got the idea of the life-prolonging qualities of yogurt from somewhere in Bulgaria, where many of the people have reportedly lived beyond the ripe old age of 100. In Soviet Georgia, where they eat yogurt as often as we eat hot dogs and hamburgers, there is a great concentration of people who have lived to be over 100 years of age. In Turkey, yogurt is primarily used as a sauce, as a bedtime snack, and it is also used to soothe an aching stomach. In many societies it is used to treat such ailments as ulcers and burns. In Persia, they think of it as a hair restorer. Mix your yogurt with some prunes and—voilá—you have a good product that will promote regularity.

Each day I come across more and more studies that are being made on the "healing" qualities of yogurt. For example, a leading medical institution in the East did some studies comparing the effect of gastric juice on yogurt and on homogenized cow's milk. They found that, " . . . the proteins in yogurt are digested more rapidly in gastric juice than are those of homogenized milk. Quantitatively it was found that yogurt is digested 1¾ times faster than milk during the first thirty minutes and a maximum of almost double the rate of digestion is reached at the one hour mark."

There are also studies being made that seem to indicate that yogurt may reduce cholesterol in the blood and may therefore help protect against atherosclerotic heart disease. Studies have further shown that yogurt may help in the rapid recovery of children who have infantile diarrhea.

Here in the United States, soft-frozen yogurt emporiums are springing up all over the place, and I think that it is a viable alternative to the hot dog stand. You will derive much more nutritional value from yogurt than from the hot dog. For this reason alone it can be a very positive new aspect in your lives. I have also noticed that a great many of these yogurt places also serve other health food products, which is another good idea.

Elise R. had imposed a debilitating reducing program on herself to take off 25 excess pounds. Most of this excess came from ice cream and bread. I switched her to my program so that she wouldn't deprive herself of needed nutrients. I gave her a whole slew of yogurt recipes and recommended that she substitute the ice cream with yogurt, and the unhealthy white bread with whole-wheat pita bread. After 6 weeks she was successful in losing her extra pounds and felt much better than she had before. Today Elise maintains her weight very well. She loves to eat in the small yogurt health food shops around town, and is more healthy for it.

At this point, I would like to give you some hints to help you stay on your feet and keep going through the day, the night, and the rest of your life. The eating pattern that I am suggesting to you is so simple that built into it is a foolproof way to stick to it. You see, I am not advocating a drastic change in your eating pattern. I am not asking you to fast, although that isn't a bad idea. Fasting for a couple of days of a month gives the body a chance to clean out and recharge itself. I am not asking you to eat only 10 grams of protein foods per day. I am not asking you to cut out all carbohydrates and drink all the water you can each day. I am only asking you to eat normal, healthy meals.

USING THIS FOOD IN AN EATING PLAN

What I am asking you to do is to use common sense and moderation. I am asking you to eat nutritiously balanced meals and to get plenty of exercise and rest. I am asking you to work towards a mentally and physically fit body. I have tried to show you the way that I and quite a number of my friends and students do it. However, within this framework there is a great deal of room for flexibility.

My eating plan is bound to keep you on your feet. If you eat nutritiously you will feel no side effects of weakness, dizziness, or the like. These side effects show up only when you go on fad diets and deprive your body of needed substances.

This is exactly what happened to a friend of mine. Horace L. was a "junk food freak" from the day he was born. He was a mama's boy, and she would stuff him full of any "junk" that her dear little child wanted any time of the day or night. This pattern stayed with him until he was a grown man. I met him while I was working in a hotel in the Catskill mountains in New York. He worked there part-time to supplement his income. We spent a lot of time together, and I used to marvel at his eating pattern. He ate the "junkiest" foods I have ever seen a person consume. Actually, I don't think that he ever had a balanced meal except when the hotel provided it for him. He would often give up a free meal at the hotel to go out and have hot dogs, french fries, and the like. It took a long, long time to bring him around to my way of thinking.

This came about after he had a rather long sick spell. It seems that his poor eating habits had finally caught up with him because his body was weak and limp, with no energy whatsoever. Fortunately I was able to help him back to health by planning some healthy meals for him—he didn't have the energy to go to a fast-food chain for his "nourishment." I also persuaded him to do some modified exercises to help his body get into shape and good health. Previously the only exercise he did was lifting his hands to his mouth to stuff it with "junk" food.

All my help made him much healthier and happier. He's always telling me how irresponsible he had been in his eating habits and how sorry he was for not following my advice sooner. My usual retort to him was "Better late than never." These days, instead of taking a "strawberry ice cream bonanza break," he takes a healthy, refreshing "yogurt break."

You can use yogurt to help you stay on your feet. I find that it is a great "pick me up" snack. It is nutritionally valuable, as I will show you later on in this chapter, and it is much healthier by far than a bag of salty, greasy potato chips. Used as an integral part of your eating pattern, yogurt can be fun.

If your palate can take the plain tart flavor of yogurt, then by all means use the plain yogurt. If you want to break into the yogurt habit gradually, try some ready-made flavored yogurts which have more calories than the plain yogurt. What I do is use a great deal of fresh fruit chopped up in plain yogurt. You have the option of doing with it what you like, but please stay away from the artificial sweeteners that are used by some yogurt manufacturers. You can experiment with various mixtures to be added to the plain yogurt. Further on in this chapter I have listed 25 ways to do this. You can add just about anything to it to make a variety of easily digestible snacks.

It is said that the protein in yogurt is digested twice as quickly as that in milk because it is partly broken down during its manufacture. I also find it a great substitute for sour cream. Try substituting yogurt for sour cream in your recipes; however, you will find that you must adjust the recipes somewhat. Yogurt also helps to keep chicken and meats very moist and succulent when you cover them with it and bake them in the oven.

Yogurt is not a complete food, so I am not advocating that you go on a yogurt binge. What I am trying to do is to make you aware of the nutritional value of the product. I am not advocating another fad diet for you. I would like you to incorporate yogurt into your eating pattern on a daily basis, but do not make it the end-all and be-all of your eating habits. Furthermore, you should always check with your doctor before changing your eating habits drastically. Yogurt is an easily digested food that is chock full of protein and calcium and should not be dismissed lightly.

Here is the nutrition information per 8 oz. cup serving of Dannon Yogurt:

	Plain Yogurt	Flavored Yogurt (coffee, lemon, vanilla)	Fruit Yogurt
Calories	150	200	260
Protein	12 grams	12 grams	10 grams
Carbohydrate	17 grams	32 grams	49 grams
Fat	4 grams (1.6%)	3 grams (1.4%)	2 grams (1.0%)

Percentage of U.S. Recommended Daily Allowances (U.S. RDA)

	Plain Yogurt	Flavored Yogurt	Fruit Yogurt
Protein	30	25	20
Vitamin A	2	2	*
Vitamin C	*	*	*
Thiamine	4	4	2

Riboflavin	30	25	20
Niacin	*	*	*
Calcium	40	40	35
Iron	*	*	*
Vitamin B$_6$	4	4	2
Vitamin B$_{12}$	20	20	15
Phosphorus	35	30	25
Magnesium	10	10	10
Zinc	8	8	6
Pantothenic Acid	10	8	6

*Contains less than 2% of the U.S. RDA of these nutrients.

The number of nutrients in this little cup fascinates me. The Dannon Yogurt Company sent me this chart in which they list the following information about the major nutrients in their product:

Protein —Builds body cells, necessary to maintain life.

Vitamin A —Promotes normal growth, especially needed for healthy eyes, skin, and mucous membranes.

Vitamin C —Helps keep blood vessels strong and develops connective tissue; also helps keep bones and teeth healthy and aids in healing wounds.

Thiamine, Riboflavin, Niacin and Vitamin B$_{12}$ —All members of the vitamin B family; help with the proper functioning of nerves, normal appetite, good digestion, and healthy skin.

Calcium and Phosphorus —Combine to help build strong bones and teeth; calcium is also important in producing healthy blood.

Iron —Required for making the oxygen-carrying cells of blood and keeping the body generally healthy.

Now, with all this information in mind, is it any wonder that I am asking you to supplement your eating with yogurt whenever you can? Instead of reaching for that candy bar, reach for a plain yogurt. I find that the fruit yogurts are a little too rich for my eating pattern. The fruit preserves are too rich in carbohydrates. This should be kept in mind when you reach for them. Don't overdo it.

Yogurt is very nutritious as a snack or a dessert. It tastes like frozen custard with a mild tang to it. The benefit that you will derive from it depends on how you introduce it into your eating pattern. Don't plan to replace all your other foods with yogurt. A sensible introduction of this product into your daily routine would be the thing to do. I have included in this chapter some rather easy recipes for your convenience. As they say, "Try them, you will like them."

HOW YOU CAN CHANGE THE FLAVOR

You can make yogurt from any kind of milk—raw, goat, sheep, and others. It is made by culturing milk with bacteria cultures, chief among which is one called *lactobacillus bulgaricus*. I have included a recipe for making yogurt, but if you're not so inclined be sure to check the label of store-bought yogurt for artificial flavoring and additives. Buy yogurt that is fresh and has no artificial ingredients. Plain yogurt is the best for you, but if you don't like plain yogurt, here are 25 quick and easy ideas for a new flavor interest, courtesy of the Dannon Yogurt Company. All add only about 25 calories or less to the 150 calories in plain yogurt.

> 2 teaspoons frozen fruit juice concentrate (orange, lemon-lime, pineapple, etc.)
> 1 teaspoon sweetened soft drink mix
> 1 teaspoon flavored gelatin dessert powder
> 1 teaspoon instant cocoa or carob powder
> 1 teaspoon pudding mix
> 1 teaspoon instant pre-sweetened tea
> 1 teaspoon maple syrup
> 1 teaspoon sugar and dash of fresh lemon or lime juice
> 1 teaspoon chocolate or carob syrup
> 1 tablespoon applesauce and dash of cinnamon
> 1 tablespoon sweetened coconut flakes
> 1 teaspoon dietetic preserves or marmalade
> 1 tablespoon canned nectar (pear, peach, apricot, and others)
> 1 tablespoon liqueur (Curacao, creme de menthe or cacao, for example)
>
> *Note:* The seasonings above are on the sweet side. These are non-sweet:
>
> 1 teaspoon instant onion soup mix or other soup mix
> 1 packet instant vegetable broth mix

1 tablespoon relish (frankfurter or hamburger)
1 teaspoon tartar sauce
1 teaspoon each catsup and brown sugar
½ teaspoon each prepared mustard and sugar
1 tablespoon each minced clams and dried chopped chives
1 tablespoon canned deviled ham
1 tablespoon mashed canned tuna fish
2 tablespoons cottage cheese
1 tablespoon each grated parmesan or romano cheese and catsup

AN ORIENTAL DANCER'S BEAUTY SECRET

We have talked about the benefits of taking yogurt internally. Now let me tell you about the benefits of applying it to your skin. No magical things are going to occur, it is not the creams that you put on that help the skin, but the massage of the application that stimulates the underlying muscles. This yogurt facial is strictly my own idea. I love it, and now I would like to share it with you. Just the other day I walked into a drug store and—what to my surprise—there I saw a facial cream with yogurt in it. I could hardly believe that someone had finally introduced yogurt for use on the face. I had just been puttering around with the idea at home rather than using prepared products.

There are varying types of treatments for all sorts of skin types. I find that a yogurt facial is a neutralizing sort of facial. It's good for all types of skin, but of course you should always check with your regular doctor or your dermatologist, if you have one, to see whether this kind of treatment will benefit your skin type. It is always good to give yourself the blotch test before you go spreading it all over your face. Put a little dab on your skin and watch your reaction to it. If any unusual blotches or other forms of reaction appear, stop the process immediately.

You will need the following materials to do your facial:

1. Gauze strips
2. Cleansing tissues
3. Cotton
4. Clean towels
5. Cold cream
6. Non-alcoholic skin toning lotion
7. Spatula for removing yogurt mixture
8. Fine table salt

A good time to have your facial would be on the weekend when you have a lot of free time. Before you start your facial make sure that your hands are very clean, because you do not want to be rubbing impurities into your skin. Listed below are the movements that you should follow when cleansing and applying creams to your face:

1. Start at the corners of your mouth and work your fingers out and up towards your ears.
2. Go up and out over your cheeks.
3. Start in the middle of your forehead, over your nose, and work your fingers out to the temples and around your eyes.
4. Go down your nose, around your mouth, and down over your chin.
5. Go down your neck and out to your shoulders.
6. Go down from your hairline at the back of your neck, down your neck to the center of your back.
7. Go out to the back of your shoulders.

There are several "recipes" that I use for my yogurt facials. Listed here are four of them:

1. I just use the plain yogurt mixture and spread it lavishly over my entire face and neck.
2. I add two teaspoons of finely grated cucumber to two tablespoons of yogurt.
3. I mix a teaspoon of honey with two tablespoons of yogurt.
4. I mix an egg yolk into two tablespoons of yogurt.

These yogurt creams are very cooling and soothing, and they will make your face tingle with freshness and smoothness. Here are the steps you should follow in your facial treatment:

1. Cleanse your face thoroughly with your favorite cleansing cream, using the movements suggested above.
2. Dip some cotton in water and squeeze it dry, then dip it in table salt and apply to your face using the movements suggested above.
3. Apply yogurt cream and let it stay on your face for about half an hour.
4. Remove mixture with a spatula and wipe the remaining mix off with tissues.

5. Apply some toning lotion with cotton, using the movements suggested above.
6. Wipe face with tissues.
7. Rinse face with warm water, then dash on some cold water.
8. Apply moisturizing lotion.
9. Apply foundation base.
10. Apply makeup if you so desire.

A good idea would be to apply your facial, then soak yourself in a good hot bath and relax all your cares away. After the facial, rinse your body with cold water. Now your body will be tingling like your face.

HOW CATHY O. CONQUERED SLUGGISHNESS

Before I get into the recipes I must tell you the story of Cathy O., who complained about sluggishness and muscle pains. She was a secretary and her job was for the most part sedentary, except for bending down to get the Z files. Her breaks were spent drinking coffee and eating sweets. I got her interested in Oriental dancing and in taking yogurt breaks, and now she is supple and motivated and I no longer hear her complaining about lack of energy or pains. She told me that she lost 6 pounds during one week of my eating pattern and exercises.

EASY RECIPES TO KEEP
YOUR FAMILY HEALTHY

Listed here are some recipes that have yogurt as an integral part of them. Have fun preparing them.

Yogurt   **yields 2 quarts**

2 quarts milk
1 cup yogurt (store bought—make sure the brand you buy has live cultures)

1. Bring milk to boil in saucepan.
2. Simmer approximately 15 minutes.

3. Remove from fire and set aside until warm (so you can comfortably place your finger in it for a few seconds).
4. Pour milk into a bowl.
5. Thoroughly mix in 1 cup yogurt.
6. Cover bowl with clean cheesecloth.
7. Wrap bowl with a heavy towel and place in a warm place for approximately 3 to 5 hours where it will not be disturbed.
8. Remove towel and cheesecloth; mixture will be firm.
9. Allow to cool and then refrigerate.

Yogurt Party Dip   yields 2 cups

2 cups yogurt
1 package onion soup mix

---

1. Mix ingredients together.
2. Place in cheesecloth and let drain for ½ hour or thereabouts.
3. Serve with pita bread or your favorite wheat cracker.

Spinach and Yogurt Appetizer   serves 4

Recipe from *The Best Foods of Russia*, copyright
© 1976 by Sonia Uvezian; reprinted by permission of Harcourt Brace Jovanovich, Inc.

1 pound spinach, washed, drained, stemmed, and coarsely chopped
½ cup water
1 small onion, finely chopped
1 cup plain yogurt
1 small clove garlic, crushed, or to taste
½ teaspoon crushed dried mint
Salt and freshly ground black pepper to taste
2 tablespoons finely chopped toasted walnuts

---

1. In a heavy saucepan combine the spinach with the water and bring to a boil over high heat.
2. Reduce the heat to low, cover, and simmer 10 minutes.
3. Drain and squeeze the spinach dry.
4. In a heavy skillet heat the oil over moderate flame. Add the onion and sauté until golden, stirring frequently.
5. Add the spinach and sauté a few minutes.

6. Remove from the heat.
7. In a mixing bowl combine the yogurt, garlic, mint, and salt and pepper until well blended.
8. Gradually stir in the contents of the skillet and mix thoroughly.
9. Taste for seasoning.
10. Transfer to a serving bowl, cover, and chill.
11. Serve sprinkled with the walnuts.

Hot Yogurt Soup with Meatballs   serves 4

Recipe from *The Best Foods of Russia*, copyright
© 1976 by Sonia Uvezian; reprinted by permission of Harcourt Brace Jovanovich, Inc.

½ pound lean beef or lamb, ground twice
1 small onion, grated
Salt and freshly ground black pepper to taste
3 cups plain yogurt
1 tablespoon flour
3½ cups beef or lamb broth
¼ cup uncooked long-grain white rice
½ cup drained canned chick-peas, rinsed
1½ cups chopped spinach leaves, or a combination of sorrel and spinach
3 to 4 tablespoons finely chopped fresh coriander leaves or parsley
3 to 4 tablespoons finely chopped dill
3 to 4 tablespoons finely chopped chives or scallions, including 2 inches of the green tops

---

1. In a mixing bowl combine the meat, onion, and salt and pepper.
2. Knead with your hands until well blended. Taste for seasoning.
3. Form the mixture into balls about 1 inch in diameter and set aside.
4. Pour the yogurt into a large, heavy pot.
5. Using a whisk or fork, beat in the flour and then the broth until well blended.
6. Season with salt and pepper.
7. Bring slowly to a boil, stirring constantly in one direction.
8. When the mixture is thickened slightly, add the meatballs and rice and simmer 10 minutes, stirring frequently.

9. Add the chick-peas and spinach and simmer about 10 minutes, or until the meatballs and rice are tender.
10. Stir in the remaining ingredients and taste for seasoning.
11. Cook 5 minutes and serve hot.

Chilled Yogurt Soup   serves 4

1 medium cucumber
2 cups plain yogurt
1 cup ice water
½ pound cold boiled lean beef, cubed
4 finely chopped scallions, including 2 inches of the green tops
2 hard-cooked eggs, chopped
2 tablespoons finely chopped fresh coriander leaves or parsley
¼ cup finely chopped fresh dill
Salt to taste

1. Peel the cucumber and halve lengthwise.
2. Cut out the seeds if too large and discard.
3. Slice the cucumber crosswise into ¼ inch pieces and set aside.
4. Pour the yogurt into a deep bowl and stir until smooth.
5. Add the ice water and mix until well blended.
6. Add the reserved cucumber pieces and the remaining ingredients.
7. Mix gently but thoroughly.
8. Taste for seasoning.
9. Serve chilled.

Spinach and Egg Salad with Yogurt   serves 4

4 cups spinach leaves
2 to 6 scallions, finely chopped, including 2 inches of the green tops

1 cup plain yogurt
½ cup olive oil
Salt and freshly ground black pepper to taste
4 hard-cooked eggs, chopped
12 black olives

1. Wash the spinach thoroughly and drain.
2. Dry with paper towels.
3. Shred and combine with the scallions in a salad bowl.
4. Beat the yogurt, olive oil, and salt and pepper with a fork until well blended.
5. Add the eggs.
6. Pour the mixture over the spinach.
7. Mix gently but thoroughly, taking care not to mash the eggs.
8. Taste for seasoning.
9. Garnish with olives.
10. Serve chilled.

Vegetable Yogurt Salad   serves 4

3 stalks celery (chopped in 1 inch cubes)
½ bunch radishes (sliced thinly)
2 green peppers (chopped)
1 cup plain yogurt
1 teaspoon mayonnaise
salt and pepper to taste
1 dozen plum tomatoes (sliced in half)

1. Mix vegetables together in salad bowl.
2. Mix mayonnaise and yogurt together well.
3. Add to vegetables and mix well.
4. Top with plum tomatoes.
5. Refrigerate until ready to serve.

Zucchini Yogurt Salad—Turkish   serves 4

3 zucchini (coarsely chopped)
¼ cup water
2 tablespoons polyunsaturated margarine

1 cup plain yogurt
1 teaspoon garlic powder
¼ teaspoon parsley
½ teaspoon mint leaves (dried)
1 teaspoon vinegar
salt and pepper to taste
1 teaspoon paprika

---

1. Place zucchini, water, and margarine in saucepan.
2. Steam until all water is absorbed.
3. Remove from heat and let cool.
4. Add yogurt, garlic, parsley, mint, and vinegar.
5. Mix well and set aside to cool.
6. Sprinkle paprika on top.
7. Refrigerate and serve cold.

Caraway Yogurt Cheese   yields 2 cups

8 cups plain yogurt
½ cup caraway seeds
salt to taste

---

1. Put yogurt in cheesecloth (approximately 24″ × 24″) with caraway seeds.
2. Tie ends into knot at top; hang it over a counter out of the way.
3. Place pan underneath to catch liquid.
4. Leave overnight.
5. Yogurt becomes hard.
6. Remove cheese and place in serving dish.
7. Add salt to taste.
8. Spread on Arabic bread and serve.

Yogurt Balls—Arabic   serves 6

yogurt cheese (see recipe)
1 cup olive oil

1. Take some yogurt cheese and make into yogurt balls (about 1½" in diameter).
2. Put in a dish and let stand several hours in refrigerator until yogurt becomes hard.
3. Put in a deep bowl.
4. Add olive oil to coat balls.
6. Stuff into Arabic bread and serve.

Yogurt and Eggs (Çilbir)—Turkish   serves 4

1 teaspoon garlic powder
2 cups yogurt
4 eggs
3 cups water
½ tablespoon vinegar
2 tablespoons butter
1 teaspoon paprika
salt and pepper to taste

---

1. Place yogurt and garlic powder in a saucepan over low flame and warm.
2. Poach eggs in water and vinegar, then drain them.
3. Place eggs on serving plate.
4. Pour yogurt on top of eggs.
5. Heat butter, add paprika and salt and pepper; simmer about 2 minutes.
6. Pour over eggs and yogurt.
7. Serve immediately.

Yogurt and Rice—Arabic   serves 4

2 cups water
3 cups yogurt
1 cup rice
1 tablespoon flour

salt and pepper to taste
¼ teaspoon paprika

---

1. Parboil rice in a deep saucepan for about ½ hour until most of the water is absorbed.
2. Drain off excess water and set rice aside.
3. Mix the flour, salt and pepper with 2 tablespoons water until a paste is formed.
4. Add this to the yogurt.
5. Then add rice and simmer for about 5 minutes.
6. Sprinkle paprika on top.

Tomato Rarebit or Fondue   serves 6

Recipe courtesy of Dannon Yogurt
and Angostura.

1 can (10¾ oz.) condensed tomato soup
1 cup plain yogurt
1 package (8 oz.) sharp cheddar cheese, grated
1 tablespoon Angostura aromatic bitters
salt and pepper to taste

---

1. In a saucepan combine all ingredients and stir over low heat until smooth and bubbling.
2. Season to taste with salt and pepper.
3. Serve hot over toast points or small hot split biscuits.
4. Can also be used as a fondue—keep hot over a warmer and spear cubes of bread, shrimp, cubes of ham, chicken or turkey, or meatballs for dipping.

Baked Macaroni and Tuna   serves 6

Recipe courtesy of Dannon Yogurt
and Angostura.

1½ cups uncooked elbow macaroni
¼ cup polyunsaturated margarine
1 large onion, chopped

1 green pepper, chopped
1 teaspoon salt
¼ teaspoon pepper
2 cups plain yogurt
2 cans (6½ oz. ea.) tuna, drained and flaked
1 can (10¾ oz.) condensed cream of celery soup
2 teaspoons Angostura aromatic bitters
1 package (8 oz.) sharp cheddar cheese, shredded

---

1. In a saucepan, cook macaroni according to package directions until tender, then drain.
2. In a small skillet, heat margarine and sauté onion and green pepper until golden.
3. In a large bowl, mix macaroni, sautéed vegetables and their drippings, and remaining ingredients.
4. Pour into well-buttered 2 quart casserole.
5. Bake in a preheated moderate oven (350° F) for 45 minutes.

Yogurt Kebab—Turkish   serves 4 or 5

1½ lbs. lamb or beef (cut into 1″ cubes)
2 tablespoons polyunsaturated oil
1 large onion (finely chopped)
1 teaspoon thyme (powdered)
¼ teaspoon parsley
2 tablespoons lemon juice
salt and pepper to taste
4 skewers
4 cups yogurt
1 teaspoon garlic powder
2 large tomatoes
4 tablespoons butter
4 pita breads
1 teaspoon paprika

---

1. Marinate meat, oil, onion, thyme, parsley, lemon juice, salt and pepper in bowl overnight in refrigerator.
2. Next day put meat on skewers.
3. Broil kebabs over charcoal or in the oven until golden brown (approx. ½ hour).

4. Place yogurt in bowl with garlic powder; put aside.
5. Peel and chop tomatoes and simmer for about 5 minutes in 2 tablespoons butter.
6. Toast both sides of pita bread and place on warmed serving dish.
7. Cut in quarters.
8. Pour cooked tomatoes over pita bread.
9. Pour yogurt sauce on top of tomatoes.
10. Place skewer of meat over sauce.
11. Place paprika in 2 remaining teaspoons of butter and simmer 2 minutes.
12. Add paprika mixture on top of meat.
13. Serve immediately.

Yogurt Soup—Turkish   serves 4

½ cup barley (optional)
4 cups chicken or beef broth
1 large onion (chopped)
3 tablespoons butter
¼ cup fresh parsley (chopped)
¼ teaspoon thyme
1 tablespoon fresh mint (chopped)
3 cups yogurt
salt and pepper to taste

1. Soak barley overnight.
2. Drain barley and place in chicken or beef broth.
3. Sauté onion in butter until lightly brown and add to barley mix.
4. Add parsley, thyme, mint, salt and pepper to onion mix.
5. Simmer on low heat for ¾ hour.
6. Just before serving, mix in yogurt thoroughly (stir yogurt well previously).
7. Serve in warm bowls.

Yogurt Sauce—Turkish   yields 1 cup

1 cup plain yogurt
1 teaspoon garlic powder
salt to taste

1. Beat all ingredients together for 5 minutes.
2. Serve on vegetables; e.g., fried eggplant, zucchini, carrots.

Yogurt Sauce (sweet)—Turkish   yields 1 cup

1 cup plain yogurt
3 tablespoons honey

---

1. Beat ingredients together for 5 minutes.
2. Serve on fresh fruits; e.g., strawberries.

Mint and Garlic Dressing   yields 3½ cups

1 tablespoon flour
2 tablespoons water
4 cups yogurt
1 tablespoon dried mint
1 teaspoon garlic powder
salt and pepper to taste

---

1. Mix flour and water to make paste in a saucepan.
2. Add yogurt and boil over low flame, stirring at intervals.
3. Add dried mint and garlic powder.
4. Serve on your favorite vegetable.

For variety—If you wish, you could substitute about ⅛ teaspoon Tabasco sauce instead of garlic powder.

Olive Dressing   yields 1⅓ cups

Recipe courtesy of Dannon Yogurt.
Used with the permission of CPC International Inc.

⅓ cup Hellmann's Real Mayonnaise
2 tablespoons finely chopped pimento-stuffed olives

2 tablespoons chopped onion
1 tablespoon chopped pimento
⅛ teaspoon garlic powder
½ teaspoon sugar (I substitute this with honey)
1 cup plain yogurt

-----

1. In a small bowl, mix mayonnaise with olives, onion, pimento, garlic powder, and honey.
2. Fold in yogurt.
3. Cover and chill until serving time.
4. Serve with salad greens, raw vegetables as a dip, or as a sandwich spread (in place of butter).

Thousand Island Dressing   yields 1⅔ cups

Recipe courtesy of Dannon Yogurt.
Used with the permission of CPC International Inc.

⅓ cup Hellmann's Real Mayonnaise
¼ cup chili sauce
2 tablespoons chopped pimento-stuffed olives
1 tablespoon chopped onion
1 tablespoon chopped green pepper
2 teaspoons chopped parsley
1 cup plain yogurt

-----

1. In a small bowl, mix mayonnaise with chili sauce, olives, onion, green pepper, and parsley.
2. Fold in yogurt.
3. Cover and chill until serving time.
4. Serve as a dressing for salad greens or as a sandwich spread (in place of butter).

Blue Cheese Dressing   yields 1½ cups

Recipe courtesy of Dannon Yogurt.
Used with the permission of CPC International Inc.

⅓ cup Hellmann's Real Mayonnaise
⅓ cup crumbled blue cheese
1 cup plain yogurt

1. In a small bowl, mix mayonnaise and blue cheese.
2. Fold in yogurt.
3. Cover and chill until serving time.
4. Serve with salad greens or with raw vegetables as a dip.

Herb Garlic Dressing   yields 1⅓ cups

Recipe courtesy of Dannon Yogurt.
Used with the permission of CPC International Inc.

⅓ cup Hellmann's Real Mayonnaise
1 teaspoon sugar (I substitute honey)
¾ teaspoon chopped chives
½ teaspoon basil leaves
½ teaspoon garlic powder
½ teaspoon oregano leaves
1 cup plain yogurt

1. In a small bowl, mix mayonnaise with honey, chives, and seasonings
2. Fold in yogurt.
3. Cover and chill until serving time.
4. Serve as a dressing for salad greens or cold cooked vegetables, spoon over sliced tomatoes just before serving, or serve as a sauce for beef fondue.

Cucumber Drink (Cacik)—Turkish   yields 3 cups

2 large cucumbers
2 cups plain yogurt
½ cup cold water
1 teaspoon garlic powder
1 teaspoon chopped dill
salt to taste

1. Peel cucumbers; chop very fine.
2. Place all ingredients in a blender or mix with mixer until a thick
   liquid is formed.
3. Refrigerate.
4. Serve in chilled glasses.
5. If you wish, you may substitute fresh mint for the dill.

Borani—a Pakistani Cocktail   yields 1½ quarts

2 cups yogurt
1 quart water
10 strips lemon peel
⅛ teaspoon chili powder
½ teaspoon fresh mint, chopped
salt and pepper to taste

1. Combine all ingredients and mix thoroughly in a cocktail
   shaker or blender.
2. Refrigerate until ready to serve.
3. Serve in chilled cocktail glasses.

Yogurt Fruit Drink   serves 2

1 cup plain yogurt
3 large fresh peaches (skinned optional)

½ cup water

---

1. Take pits out of peaches.
2. Put above ingredients in blender and blend until peach has dissolved.
3. This is best if you drink it immediately while foam is still on top.

Any fresh fruit can add variety to this recipe.

Pineapple Orange Shake   serves 4

**Recipe courtesy of Dannon Yogurt
and Angostura**

2 eggs
2 cups pineapple-orange yogurt
1 cup milk
1 teaspoon Angostura aromatic bitters

---

1. Combine all ingredients in a blender and whirl at top speed until smooth.
2. Serve in tall glasses poured over crushed ice.

Pineapple-Orange Thick Shake   serves 8

**Recipe courtesy of Dannon Yogurt
and Angostura**

2 eggs
1 cup crushed pineapple
1 cup instant non-fat dry milk
2 cups plain yogurt
1 can (6 oz.) frozen concentrated orange juice
2 teaspoons Angostura aromatic bitters
2 tablespoons sugar (I substitute honey)

1. Combine all ingredients in a blender and whirl at top speed until smooth.
2. Serve in tall glasses poured over crushed ice.

Yogurt and Fruit Gel   serves 6

1 package gelatin (any fruit flavor)
1 cup hot water
1 cup yogurt (vanilla, lemon, or coffee flavored)
1 cup mixed fresh fruit

1. Mix gelatin with hot water until powder is dissolved.
2. Add yogurt and mix ingredients together (stir yogurt previously).
3. Pour into gelatin mold and place in refrigerator until mixture thickens.
4. Serve cold.

Dannon Yogurt Pie   serves 8

Recipe courtesy of Dannon Yogurt
A recipe developed by Pearl Byrd Foster

1 tablespoon unflavored gelatin
¼ cup cold water
2 egg yolks, slightly beaten
¼ cup milk
2 cups vanilla yogurt
1 teaspoon vanilla
8 ounces Neuchatel cheese (room temp.) (If Neuchatel cheese is not available, use 16 oz. of cream cheese).
8 ounces cream cheese (room temp.)
1 teaspoon molasses
1 tablespoon clover honey
½ cup graham cracker crumbs
1 graham cracker crumb shell

1. Soften gelatin in cold water and dissolve over hot water.
2. Add milk to the slightly beaten egg yolks and cook with the gelatin over gently boiling water until it coats a silver spoon, then set aside to cool.
3. Cream the cheese, vanilla, molasses, and honey together and add one cup of yogurt; continue to cream until smooth.
4. Pour the cold gelatin mixture slowly over the cheese, stirring constantly.
5. Add the second cup of yogurt and mix well.
6. Pour into baked graham cracker crumb shell and chill until firm.
7. When ready to serve, sprinkle top with graham cracker crumbs to make 1 (10") pie.

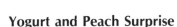

Yogurt and Peach Surprise   serves 6

1 lb. fresh peaches
2 jars strained peaches (baby food)
1 cup yogurt (vanilla or any other flavor)
½ cup fresh walnuts (shelled and chopped fine)

1. Cut fresh peaches into cubes.
2. Mix strained peaches and yogurt.
3. Cover fresh peach mixture with yogurt mixture.
4. Top with walnuts.
5. Serve.

Chapter

10

an arabian nights
entertainment

When you hear the words "Arabian Nights Entertainment" you immediately think of some exotic Middle Eastern setting complete with sultans, dancing girls, wines, and so forth, don't you? That's exactly the kind of atmosphere I want you to create at your party. The party at which you are going to be the center of attraction with your new shape is going to be your "coming out" party. You are going to shine and radiate before your guests' very eyes. Your party can take on an Arabic, Turkish, or Greek flavor. Though these various cultures overlap in many ways, there are also definite differences that make each one a unique entity. You could compare them to your family of children: they are all yours; however, each child has his or her own unique personality that differentiates him or her from the rest. That's how I like to look at the Middle East and its environs. Depending on which culture you choose, you would decorate your apartment in the appropriate corresponding decor, complete with typical foods of the particular country.

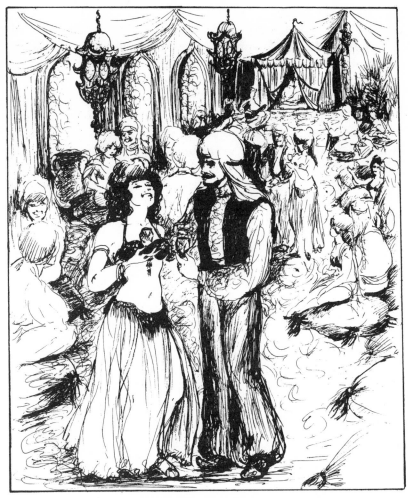

Arabian Nights Party

A Brief Historical Background of Oriental Dance

When one thinks of the Middle East today, the things that come to mind are the wars between the Arabs and Israelis, camels, deserts, the Suez Canal, oil sheiks and oil, and oil, and more oil. These things are an integral part of this region. However, we could also think of its ancient history when it was the cradle of civilization. We could also think of the three great monotheistic religions that were started there: Judaism, Christianity, and Islam.

The Ottoman Turks in about 1350 took over the whole region from Romania to Greece. They occupied Constantinople (modern Istanbul) in 1453. Beginning in 1699 the Ottoman Empire started to fall apart, and finally in 1923 the Turkish Republic was promulgated under Mustapha Kemal (Ataturk). Under Ataturk's rule there were many firsts. It was the first time that any Moslem country had separated government and religion. It was Ataturk who took the veils off of the women and had them come out of the harems. Entertainment, especially in the harems, had included Oriental dances. Sultans and caliphs enjoyed the dancing girls. In more recent times these dances were performed in cafes.

The dances of Ancient Egypt were varied in nature. Some of them were done in worship to the sun, some were astronomical dances and many centered around the dead.

The Oriental dance is not typical of the ancient Greek world, though they have adopted it for their restaurants and night clubs here in the United States. Occasionally the modern Greeks will have an Oriental dancer appear at their festive occasions, but it is not the usual custom. Today the Greeks are dancing more of their traditional circle folk dances. In ancient Greece their entertainment took the form of outdoor dramatic performances of tragedies, choral hymns, and dramatic dances.

How to Turn Your House
Into a Middle Eastern Fantasyland

Well, seven weeks are up and you are going to create these ancient settings in your home or wherever you have chosen to have a fantastic, exciting, exotic, and titillating evening. If you are going to give this gala event in your home, then get your tent ready. If this indoor tent idea sounds "far out," well, have I got news for you, it's not as far out as you think. Go to your nearest party store and you'll find a small tent that you can place in a strategic spot in your home. This is one piece of ingenuity guaranteed to blow your friends' minds, next to seeing you in all your glory parading your new shape in your Oriental dance costume. If you can, move all your furniture to another room and use large throw pillows for your guests instead of chairs.

If you can afford it and have the space, another possibility is for you to rent a very large tent and set that up in your back yard. If you don't have a back yard but have some vacant land lying dormant and unused somewhere, then pitch your tent there. Think of the possibilities—you could invite a few close friends to visit you for the weekend, have them sleep under the stars, get some good, clean fresh air, get some togetherness, and when the moment was right, you could whip out your Middle Eastern records and battery-run record player (or else you could use tapes) and turn into the beautiful dancing girl of the Nile right before their shocked eyes.

Of course you will have to take a lot of things with you to that empty lot in the country, but it will be worth it, believe me. The meze (hors d'oeuvres) could be left at a friend's house until you are ready to use them, or if you are resourceful, you could get a portable refrigerator unit. These are relatively inexpensive, and you can get some dry ice to do an effective refrigeration job.

So those are your three possibilities: convert your house, your backyard, or your vacant lot into an Arabian wonderland. Start by making a list of all the things that will make this night a success. First I'll give you some ideas for the Middle Eastern theme. Here are some things that you must keep in mind:

1. Middle Eastern decor—rugs, lamps, throw pillows, canopy, furniture, and other knickknacks
2. Guest list and invitations
3. Costume for your beautiful "new" body
4. Food
5. Entertainment

You should begin working out the details weeks before the party so that everything will go smoothly and you will be able to devote your time entirely to your guests. You do not want to be in the kitchen making another batch of baba ghannouj, slicing the roast lamb, or whatever. Make sure by planning ahead that you will be free to mingle and entertain your guests as you should. It's nice for your guests to meet new people, but let's face it, they also came to see you too, so it's important for you to be out of the kitchen.

Give your old Oriental rug or carpet (the distinction between the two is size—larger than approximately 6' by 9' is a carpet) a good cleaning. Perhaps you could pick up a rug and use it as a wall hanging for the occasion. Who knows, it may become a permanent fixture in your home. They do have some rather inexpensive, good-looking Oriental rugs that will fit into a small budget. Some of the Oriental dance boutiques have the most adorable rugs with Middle Eastern themes such as Oriental dancers on them.

You will need some Middle Eastern objets d'art to create an authentic atmosphere. One such object is the ancient nargeeli (water pipe). I remember seeing my grandfather puffing away at this rather strange looking object with delight. Today the young folks may find other things to put in it rather than good old Turkish tobacco.

If you do not live near a Middle Eastern shop, or if you can't afford to buy some Middle Eastern knickknacks, here are some inexpensive ideas and a few helpful hints for making simple Middle-Eastern-style items to make your party a smashing success.

Lamps

Many Middle Eastern lamps are made of brass with brightly colored stones inserted in them for the light to shine through. Many of them are also made of filigree with some beautiful handmade designs on them. Filigree is made of fine wire, usually gold, silver, or silver-gilt, which is worked into delicate, intricate designs, either of a kind of openwork or as surface decoration for a gold or silver ground to which it is soldered.

In order to get this kind of effect, first you will need some gold or silver metallic paper. Cut some very small holes in the paper, let all your creativity go to work, and think about a design before you start cutting. Remember those paper snowflakes you used to make in school? Well, you can apply the same technique to this project by folding your paper several times in order to get an even pattern. The holes should be quite small to achieve a filigree effect. I usually use a sheet of paper approximately 9″ × 14″; however, you can experiment with various sizes. In fact it would be nice to vary the sizes of your "lamps." After you have cut out your design, staple or glue the edges together so that the paper forms a round tube. Make three or four small holes at the edge, attach some string, and hang it from the ceiling. You can use heavy-duty tape for this.

Of course the most effective way to use these "lamps" would be to put them over lightbulbs so that light can shine through the openings and create an exciting pattern as it shines on the walls, ceiling, or whatever. If you do this, make sure that the paper does not rest on the bulb, and use a bulb of very low wattage to prevent the paper from burning. Experiment with different colored bulbs to achieve the ultimate in excitement.

Another alternative would be to attach the paper to an existing lamp shade so that the light will shine through. This will cut down on the amount of light you get from the lamp, but who needs a lot of light at a time like this? I always thought that dim lights added more atmosphere to a room anyway.

Canopy

You can make your own canopy with simple bed sheets. Try to get sheets that are colorful so that the ceiling will come to life. If patterned ones with an exotic design are not available, then take plain white sheets and try your hand at tie-dyeing, which is a process of folding fabric, tying, and dyeing it. If you are not familiar with the process, here is a very brief explanation. Spread the sheet on a flat surface. Grasp a section of the fabric with one hand and pull it up in a point. While holding the bunched-up cloth, wrap a cord tightly around the bunch, about six inches down from the point in a criss-cross manner. Without tying off the cord, grasp another section nearby and tie in the same manner. Continue this until the entire surface of the cloth has been bunched and tied. Dye in one color at a time, and when dry, remove the cord and tie other sections. Add different colors as you go along to make your design more interesting. Different kinds of objects can be tied into the cloth as well, each resulting in a distinctive pattern image. Pieces of wood lattice stripping, wood or plastic thread spoons are all suitable. The sheet can be tacked to the ceiling on cork that has an adhesive backing, or you could use some other form of stripping such as wood or masonite. Check your local hardware store or lumber yard for the materials suitable for your type of ceiling. I'll admit this is a rather difficult thing to do because it can be damaging to the ceiling if you do not have wooden beams exposed on your ceiling or if you do not do a thorough job. However, I wouldn't worry too much about this aspect of the decor because it can get to be a major job that you may not want to undertake. It might be an idea that you may want to introduce into a room that needs an added spark, so you can file that away for a redecorating project. If you must go about it for your party, seek outside professional help.

Throw Pillows

Some party stores rent these. If you have a sewing machine, and more importantly, if you know how to use it, you are in business! Get some heavy drapery or upholstery fabric in exotic colors. Prints or solid colors are acceptable. Exercise your color preferences here. The pillows should be square and approximately 24" x 24" when finished, so cut them 25" square to allow for a half-inch seam all around. If you have a lot of fat friends who haven't tried my exercises and eating pattern, then make them larger. Join all sides of the fabric together with a half-inch seam, leaving a small opening on one side so that you can stuff the pillow. You can use any kind of stuffing, such as scraps of fabric or chopped foam. The latter is readily available in dime and department stores. Since people will be sitting on them, it is important that they be sturdy so that they aren't flattened out by the first person who sits on them.

Furniture You Will Need

Go into the Middle Eastern or Indian stores and look for bargains. In many Middle Eastern countries, eating arrangements are usually low and close to the ground or floor. This is one of the ancient traditions of that part of the world. Of course there are also Western-style chairs, tables, sofas, and the like all over the place. However, there are still people whose only form of seating arrangement consists of throw pillows or low stools around a very low table, usually a large brass tray set on top of wooden legs. I enjoy this sort of seating because it always seems to make things cozier and more friendly.

The large brass trays, which can be used in a utilitarian manner as tables, can also be used in a purely decorative way. Their designs are very intricate and unique. They don't take up that much room because, after a meal of tea or whatever, you can just take them up and hang them on the wall or lean them up in a corner out of the way. In countries where space is so valuable and scarce this is a perfect idea. In my home I have a couple of brass trays that I use as coffee tables and I also have some hanging on the walls strictly for decorative purposes.

Guests

Try to invite those of your friends who you think would enjoy this kind of party, and if you are daring, invite a few "potentials." By this I mean people you think have possibilities for widening their horizons in terms of gaining from this experience, people you think will perk up with a little added spice in their lives. This will be your good deed for the night, and you may make some converts. I have seen many people's lives change from a simple one-time exposure to the Oriental dance.

Suggest to your friends that they wear an outfit with a Middle Eastern theme, but for heaven's sake don't bar them from the party just because they don't have the latest in kaftans from Iran, Lebanon, or Turkey. You have the option of making this a complete surprise to your friends, so in this case just invite them for a party and let them "come as they are," or you can advise that there is a theme to your party and that you would like them to dress accordingly.

For your really daring friends, ready-made Oriental dance costumes are available. Many aspiring Oriental dancers use these as practice costumes. They are reasonably priced and good for the person who does not sew. Your guests can also pick up some belledi dresses or other types of ethnic clothes at some of the more enterprising shops.

Costume

For those of you who can sew, here are a few tips for making your own Oriental dance costume. The costume consists of the following parts: bra, hip band, skirt, veil, and a few other accessories such as panty briefs. For you curious ones, yes, Oriental dancers do wear something under their skirts!

Let's start with the bra and hip band. For these you will need a brassiere that has some body to it; approximately one and a half yards of felt fabric; some sequins by the yard, assorted beads, sequins, and other trimmings that you think will add to the beauty of your costume; heavy gauge thread; dressmaker's wax. And yes, don't forget the needle! A few different sizes of needles are essential since you will need extra-fine ones for bead work and thicker ones for heavy sewing.

The Bra

1. Take a regular bra and cut off the straps and back. Use only the cups of the bra.
2. Cover the cups of the bra with felt; the felt must conform to the shape of the bra. We do this because it is much easier to sew on felt than the fabric of the bra.
3. To make the straps, cut about six 36" strips out of the felt. Double them and sew the edges together with a zigzag stitch if possible. This will make the strips stronger.
4. Attach the straps to the edges of the bra and place heavy hooks at the ends of the straps after you have measured them for fit. You can decide whether you want to make a halter effect or just have the straps go over the shoulder.

5. Wax your thread quite often so that the beads will not cut into the thread, and start decorating it.
6. Decide what design you want on your bra and go to it. I find that a lot of hanging things on the bra emphasize your movements when you dance. Actually you may sew anything on the bra to cover it in a decorative way.

The Hip Band

1. Take about half a yard of felt fabric and fold it in two.
2. Trace an outline of a hip band on the felt. The hip band may be shaped to your liking, but try not to make it wider than four inches at any spot.
3. Cut out the hip band, leaving about two inches of an overlap for heavy-duty hooks and eyes for the closing.
4. Zigzag the edges of the hip band together.
5. Sketch a design on the hip band, then sew on beads, sequins, and other trimmings. Make sure to fasten your thread properly.
6. Take a piece of dressmaker's half-inch tape the length of the hip band and sew on a three-and-a-half-inch fringe of beads. This can be done by stringing approximately twelve beads on your thread and knotting the ends securely. You place these lengths next to each other to make the fringe look full. (Fringe can be bought ready made.)
7. Attach fringe to the bottom edge of hip band.
8. Put hooks and eyes at edges to close hip band.
9. Face inside of hip band with satin fabric to give a finished look.

The Skirt

1. Buy about seven and a half yards of fabric. Any interesting printed or plain silk chiffon will be right. Brocades are nice too, but expensive.
2. Cut the skirt on the bias. This is much better than cutting it on the straight, which would save fabric but would have less movement to it. To do this, fold the fabric in three equal pieces. Find the center of the selvage side and cut out a half-moon shape. Measure the length you wish and leave about two inches for a hem.

3. Join sides of two panels with a half-inch seam. Leave one panel free for the front.
4. Put a band the size of your waist and a little more around the top of the skirt with a hook at the end to close it.
5. Hem the bottom of the skirt with a narrow hem. If you wish, put a colorful trim on the bottom of the skirt. This will enhance the look of the skirt.

> *Note:* It is important to get your skirt as even as possible. The best way to do this is to get someone to even it while you have it on. If you can't get someone to help you, hang the skirt in the doorway or on anything available and use your eye to get it as even as possible.

The Veil

1. Take from two to two and a half yards of fabric and hem the edges. This fabric can be the same as the skirt or it can be different. It depends on your taste.
2. Put some trim around the edges if you wish.

When you put all these things together you should look something like the picture shown here. You can drape your veil around you, if you wish, to be more modest as you walk around chatting with your guests.

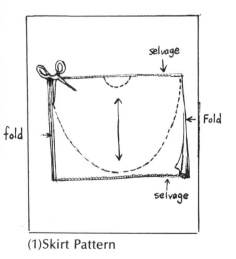

(1) Skirt Pattern

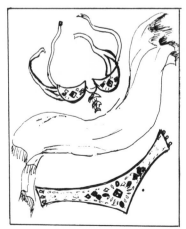

(2) Costume Parts

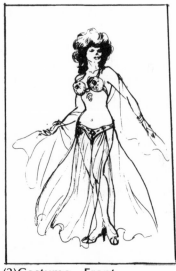 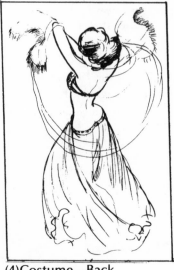

(3)Costume—Front   (4)Costume—Back

Oriental Dance Costume

Food

Sharpen your taste buds and prepare yourself for exotic treats. In Chapter 11 I've given you some of my Middle Eastern and other recipes. Use as many of these as you wish. A word of warning, though: No Middle Eastern party would be complete if you did not serve the following:

a) Hummus bi taheeni (chickpea dip)
b) Baba Ghannouj (eggplant dip)
c) Khubz (Arabic bread)—The Greeks call this pita bread. It is used instead of crackers for dips
d) Tabbouleh (mint and parsley salad)—This is a very popular Lebanese dish
e) Boerek (meat, cheese, or spinach-filled pastries)
f) Koefte (meatballs)
g) Turkish coffee

At this kind of party I would suggest that you serve a smorgasbord dinner rather than a sit-down dinner. Some buffets can be a nutrition-conscious person's nightmare. If you ever go to a regular type of party where the table is filled with a lot of "junk" food, I would suggest that you try to pick out the most nutritious-looking dish and eat that. There is no law that says you must eat everything in sight. The same thing is true with drinking. It has been a very frustrating problem to show up at someone's house and have drinks stuffed in your hands every two minutes. A great idea is to make your own drink. A glass of club soda, complete with straw and cherry, could fool the best of hostesses. Better yet, get a martini glass, fill it with water, and stick in an olive. The next thing to do is to hang onto this concoction and never let your hostess see your hands empty. If she does catch you with an empty hand and shoves a drink in it, take a sip in front of her and slip away at the first chance and get rid of it. If I must drink, I usually have one or two glasses of white wine. A favorite drink of mine is mineral spring water.

It may seem that I disapprove of alcoholic drinking, and maybe I do. I think that drinking should be done with utmost moderation, and if you can abstain, all the better. I haven't been able to find out what nutritional value there is in any hard liquor.

However, some liqueurs are great digestive aids. I would suggest you serve some raki (Turkish), ouzo (Greek), arak (Arab-Lebanon), zibib (Egyptian), or pernod (French) with your hors d'oeuvres. These are drinks that have an anisette flavor, and they are virtually alike. If you want to be really different, serve some tea or any other exotic drink in small glasses. This is the way tea is usually served in the Middle East, Turkey, and Greece.

Decorate your tables in a creative way. Maybe you would like to pick up some inexpensive ethnic flags and use them to decorate your table. You could really go to town and get flags of all the Middle Eastern countries and use them. Little camels or other Middle Eastern knickknacks are interesting objects that can fill out your table.

Make up a menu of the things that you are serving. If you can draw, sketch a little picture to go with each dish, or better yet, make some labels about 3" x 12" and put them near each dish. Secure them to the table or tablecloth so that your mischievous friends don't get at them to play some switching games on you! This may seem like an oversimplified way· of doing this; however, remember that many of your friends may not be familiar with the Middle Eastern dishes. Besides that, you don't want to be standing behind the table all night answering the inevitable question, "What's that?" Another cute idea would be to write a short description of each dish and stick them up on a nearby wall with pictures if you have them.

If you wish to go further, you can make an individual menu for each person. Take a piece of plain 8½" x 11" paper, fold it in half, and on the outside write the following information:

Title: Middle Eastern Party

Date:

Time:

Place: (include your name, address, and apartment number)

Entertainment:

On the inside you can write the menu. You have the option of giving these to the people when they are at the party, or if you wish, you could send them out in place of an invitation. If you are sending them out as an invitation, so indicate on the front. You will also have to add the expected dress of the evening. When I make the theme of the party a surprise I sometimes tack the menu and other information outside my apartment door. It is a great conversation piece, and will your friends ever be surprised! You can also tack a box of antacid tablets to the bottom of the menu to show your friends that you are very enterprising and are prepared for all eventualities, and most of all, that you have a sense of humor. You'll hear the laughter outside your door before they get a chance to ring the doorbell.

Entertainment

All you really need are some Middle Eastern records to set the mood of the evening. In the appendix you will find a list of some records and where they can be found.

Although any Middle Eastern record will do as background music, I have a few suggestions to make. There is one record that I would like to recommend for its soothing, sensual tones. It will provide an enchanting, dreamlike atmosphere to your party, and before you know it, the music will be seeping into the very bones of your guests, carrying them away on a magic carpet. Here is the record: *Music for an Arabian Night*, Ron Goodwin and His Orchestra, Capitol. Later on, when the party gets really hot, you can speed up the tempo a bit and put on some really heavy Middle Eastern music, such as:

—*The Joy of Belling Dancing*, George Abdo, Monitor
—*Ode To An Oud*, John Berberian, Mainstream. (This is a dynamic two-record set, and a truly worthwhile investment.)

—*Strictly Belly Dancing*, Eddie "The Sheik" Kochak, Scepter Records or *Ameraba* (So far there are six volumes in this series.)

The Middle Eastern party is the one that I have described in great detail. However, if you want to add a Turkish touch, that decor and food will be very similar to the Middle Eastern. You can pick up some posters on Turkey from the Turkish consulate or even from a travel agent in your city to add a more truly Turkish touch.

Listed here are a few Turkish records for your convenience:

—*Alla Turca*, Ozel, El-Ay Records
—*An Evening in Istanbul*, Capitol Records
—*Rendezvous in Istanbul*, The Gomidas Band, Roulette
—*Soraya, My Love, Songs From the Middle East*, Soraya Melik, Monitor
—*Turkish Delight*, The Dolgru Yol Turkish Ensemble, Monitor

To add a more Greek flavor you'll have to make a few changes to the Middle Eastern ideas. First of all you should ask your guests to perhaps wear togas of some sort (bed sheets make excellent togas) or some other typical Greek style of dress.

Greek decorations are in order. Get some Greek columns from your favorite party store. You could hang some grapes (fresh or artificial) around the room to give the appearance of an outdoor vineyard. You can either sit on the floor or on more conventional seating.

There are Greek record stores all over the place, and just about any record purchased there will enhance your party. Some of the more popular Greek recording artists here in the United States include the Trio Belcanto, Nana Mouskouri, and the music of the famous composer Mikis Theodorakis. Listed here are some fun Greek records that you could add to your record collection:

—*Dance the Greek Way, The Spectacular Bouzoukee of Takis*, Takis Elenis, Monitor
—*Feenjon Goes Greek*, Feenjon Group, Monitor
—*Nana Mouskouri Sings Greek Songs by Manos Hadjidakis*, Nana Mouskouri, Fontana Records
—*Recorded Live at a Greek Party*, The Hellenes, Tifton Live Sound Series

The food can be virtually the same as the Middle Eastern and Turkish; however, to make it more authentically Greek I would suggest the following menu instead:

a) Greek salad
b) Tarama (fish roe mix)
c) Pita bread or another Greek bread
d) Chunks of feta cheese
e) Small green pepper dolmas
f) Small shish kebabs (souvlakia in Greek)
g) Roast leg of lamb or moussaka
h) Spinach pie
i) Turkish coffee

I have shown you how to have a great and exciting night full of fantasy from A Thousand and One Nights (The Arabain Nights Entertainment). However, you need not confine your enjoyment to your home. Start visiting some of the Middle Eastern clubs in your city. There you can get up and dance and let your hair down in a way you hardly ever see in other nightclubs. There you can join in the singing, the dancing, the clapping of hands, and the general festiveness and joyousness that prevails in the Middle Eastern and Greek clubs. Many a night you can see quite a few of the top Oriental dancers, caught up by the music, dancing for their own enjoyment.

At most clubs there is a set orchestra; however, many nights you will see musicians from the audience join in and "jam" with the club's orchestra. Since many of these performers and musicians travel a great deal, when they come back to town they will drop into the clubs just to hang out and see old friends and catch up with the latest happenings of the day. These clubs act as meeting places for the people in the business.

Since I teach public school I don't get too much of an opportunity to travel except during my vacations. When I do travel, one of the first things I do when I get into a new town is to drop by the local Middle Eastern nightclub or Greek restaurant where they usually have an Oriental dancer. It is a good way to keep on top of what's happening in the business, and you will always meet people who have common interests.

Now that this whole new world has been opened to you, I expect that you will be doing likewise. I know that you will be entering my world often. Enjoy it and stay healthy and happy.

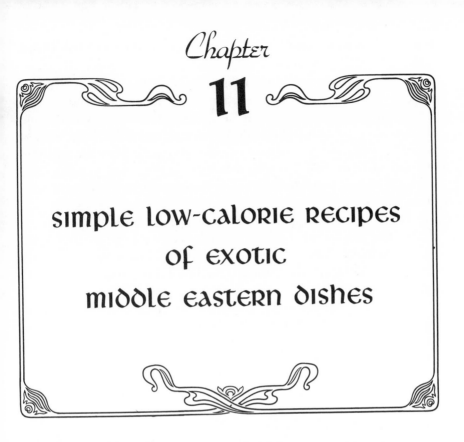

Chapter

11

simple low-calorie recipes
of exotic
middle eastern dishes

The recipes included here are some of my favorite dishes, most of which have a Middle Eastern flavor to them. I have striven to make them as simple as possible. Many of the ingredients can be found in any supermarket; however, for the more unfamiliar ingredients it would be best to visit your local Greek or Middle Eastern grocery. For your convenience, the appendix includes a short list of ethnic stores in many cities across the United States. The great thing about these recipes is that they do not include any expensive products, and they are very easy to prepare.

Alice M. will be a witness to that. Bob and Alice M. were a married couple that enjoyed dining out on a regular basis. It seems that Alice didn't like to cook, and since Bob liked to eat, this seemed like the perfect solution. I met them in a Middle Eastern restaurant in Brooklyn. They were sitting at the table next to me and my friend, and since I sensed that this was their first experience in a Middle Eastern restaurant, I tried to help them make an intelligent selection.

One thing led to another and I offered to give Alice a few of my easy Middle Eastern recipes. We also discussed the fact that they were both a little overweight. I discussed my idea for losing weight, but didn't get too much of a reaction from them that evening.

About three weeks later I got a call from Alice, who excitedly told me that she and Bob had decided that it was time for them to start eating sensibly and to begin an exercise program. They thought that my approach seemed like fun, and they were calling to get a little help. Of course I couldn't wait to get some new converts, so I gave them all the help I could.

From time to time I had to act as a morale booster. They were a challenging pair for me, because I hadn't dealt with that many couples before. Actually, I found it easier to deal with one person at a time, since one could easily discourage the other if that person wasn't making headway.

They took a little longer to lose the weight and get into a maintaining eating pattern because Bob wasn't too keen on the Oriental dance exercises, or any other type of exercise, at first. Once he got the hang of it, it was smooth sailing.

Collectively they lost 23 pounds between them in about three weeks. Two weeks after that they lost another 15 pounds. They were so excited that this worked for them that they totally immersed themselves into the Middle Eastern culture. They frequent the Greek cabarets and will get up at the downbeat of a doumbeg and dance, dance, dance. They have found a nice balance between their eating pattern and exercise routines. Instead of doing their exercises at home all the time, they make it a habit of going out to dance several times a month. I must also mention here that they are saving a great deal of money because, guess who is now cooking up a storm? Yes, Alice has become a regular galloping gourmet.

Middle Eastern cooking is very economical in that little food is ever discarded. Leftovers are always mixed with new ingredients to give them new life. Even when they start from scratch, they stretch their meats with lots of vegetables, rice, and the like. Too much meat isn't good for you anyway, and you can obtain your protein from nuts, milk, and many other products. In the Middle East, meats are terribly expensive; hence, the ingenuity of stretching what one has to make more. In ancient times the lamb was used for sacrifice because it was believed to be pure. In the Christian religion it was a symbol of Jesus Christ. Lamb is the most common meat eaten throughout the Middle East, Greece, and Turkey.

There is no one ingredient that is dominant in Middle Eastern or Turkish cuisine. The French are known for their sauces; Italians for their pasta; the Chinese for their vegetables; the Hawaiians for their poi and roast pork. Take away any of these and they lose their identity. This is not so of the Middle Eastern cuisine. It is truly a rich cuisine. There are hundreds of ways to prepare rice (pilav) or a simple vegetable like eggplant.

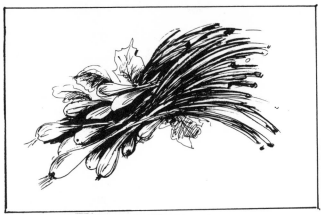

Scallions

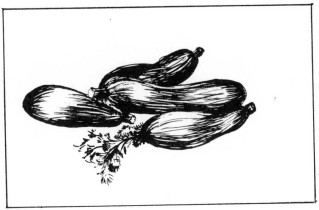

Squash

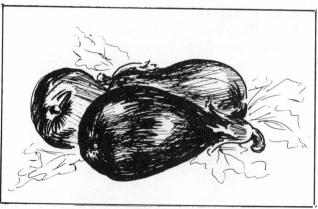

Eggplant

The Middle Easterners got their food from plants, but plants were also used for medicinal purposes. In Egypt the lotus was used for food, and it was even made into bread. The fig plays an important part in the food of the Middle East. In ancient times it was believed to be the forbidden fruit rather than the well-known apple. Some even believe it to be the tree of life as spoken about in Genesis, Chapter 2, verse 9. The pomegranate is also an important food in the Middle East.

When one thinks of the typical Middle Easterner of the older generation (around 60 years old) one thinks of a very fat old lady, bent over with age, wrapped in black from head to toe. This picture is perhaps a very accurate one; but it isn't the picture that I want you to keep in mind while reading this book. That era in the Middle East has long passed, and today we see trim women parading in the latest Givenchy and in your basic department store American-style clothing in the streets of Istanbul, Cairo, and Beirut. Needless to say, that little old lady in black pops up now and then to remind us of the past. The new generation of Middle Easterners, and indeed, more and more people all over the world, are becoming more and more aware of their bodies.

In most Middle Eastern countries the women have also been permitted to become aware of their faces—no longer do they cover them and hide them from view. You too must become aware of your body and not take it for granted. Then and only then are you going to try to do something about your body to help keep it functioning the way it must function in order to last a full lifetime free of all sorts of illnesses that can be easily prevented.

By no means am I going to ask you to take on the mentality of the Middle Easterner or their mores. You are going to preserve your own ethnic background, but you are going to become aware of a whole new section of the world. To narrow it down even further, you are going to cull some health and beauty benefits from a dance that is as ancient as time itself.

On The Flight

Jack R., for instance, really benefitted from my plan without going overboard with the Middle Eastern culture. Returning from a South American trip last year I was busy chatting with some of the passengers about the trip. As with most returning passengers, I overheard "the pledge": "I really stuffed myself on that trip. Monday morning I'm going on a diet."

Jack R. repeated "the pledge" numerous times, yet I noticed he was severely overweight. I then discovered he was a hypnotist hired by overweight and "oversmoking" people to assist them in abstinence, and yet he could not help himself.

Having just returned from Peru, I knew he had an interest in other cultures, so I began telling him about my Middle Eastern diet plan. Apparently his curiosity was piqued, and he began writing down some of my recipes. Two weeks later he called me, expressing excitement over his weight loss, and said he felt so good about himself he was ready to try the exercises.

Two months and 28 pounds passed, and "the pledge" has become a lifelong vow. Jack R. suggests the plan to many of his clients, and they are enjoying their "new selves" together.

First, let us go back a little in history and learn a bit more about the area we call the Middle East. This is essential so that you can become a well-rounded person. Many of the Oriental dancers in the United States have no roots in the Middle East, Greece, or Turkey. However, when they get involved in the dance they also get involved in the culture and everything that goes on in that part of the world. Today, Oriental dance schools are even giving workshops in front of the pyramids of ancient Egypt. When one talks of the Middle East or the Near East one thinks of Algeria, Egypt (the United Arab Republic), Iraq, Israel, Jordan, Kuwait, Lebanon, Libya, Morocco, Saudi Arabia, Sudan, Syria, Tunisia, Turkey, and Yemen. These were all countries of the Ottoman Empire at one time or the other, and that's how the Middle East is somehow tied to Turkey in my mind.

By A. D. 715 the followers of Islam had moved westward as far as Spain and eastward as far as Afghanistan, Pakistan, and India. The Arabs were everywhere by the middle of the eighth century. In 1071 the Seljuks from Turkestan conquered Asia Minor. Then the Crusades occurred. Then the Mongols under Genghis Kahn did their thing. After that the Mamluks of Egypt roamed about. By 1517 the whole eastern Mediterranean was occupied by Ottoman Turks. They ruled over this territory until the end of World War I. By the twentieth century the Ottoman Empire was known as the "sick man of Europe." And after World War I the Ottoman Empire was divided. All in all the Muslim Arabs had been under Turkish rule for over 400 years.

This is why these countries are very similar in nature even today. I am fascinated with the things that this ancient world produced: for example, the three pyramids of Giza, Egypt were built as tombs for three kings—Cheops (Khufu), Cheophren (Kheophren), and Menkaru (Mycerinus)—over 4500 years ago. The largest pyramid, Khufu, is thought of as one of the seven wonders of the ancient world. I recently visited this ancient site and was overwhelmed by its magnificence.

The ancient history of that part of the world has been quite interchangeable because it seems that each of those civilizations had a turn at conquering someone else's territory. The Persians, for example, were in Egypt at various times (fifth century B.C. and A.D. 616) and then Egypt later fell into the hands of the Arabs during the tenth century. The Greeks Alexander and Ptolemy even had their chance in Egypt too. Alexander's empire stretched far and wide, and through him Greek customs and traditions were brought to the Middle Eastern countries. Alexander the Great was king of Macedonia from 336-323 B.C., and he conquered the Greek city-states and ruled the Persian Empire from Asia Minor and Egypt to India.

Greece isn't considered part of the Middle East; however, for my purposes I have loosely linked it there because the Greek civilization was entwined with the Middle Eastern countries and there is a distinct similarity in the customs and mores. The Greeks were indeed a great civilization. They gave us the first Olympic games in 776 B.C. The greatest century for Greece was the fifth century B.C., when the temple of Zeus was built. The fantastic statue of this god was also considered one of the seven wonders of the ancient world.

The Turks were never colonized by other peoples. The modern Turks are direct descendants of the Ottoman Turks. The Ottoman

Empire lasted for about 600 years. It finally collapsed at the end of World War I. The Ottoman Empire under Suleyman the Magnificent was great between 1520-1566. After that it went downward. Turkey is one of the non-semitic countries and not considered part of the Arab world. The other non-semitic country is Iran.

In the Middle East the kitchen is the center of the woman's home. It is here that she is the mistress of the house, and she wields her mastery over foods by preparing an appetizing list of one dish more delicious and exotic than the other. Even in the poorest of homes there is a variety of meals prepared.

Food has a lot of significance in that part of the world. They have an abundance of dishes that are eaten at certain times of the year. For instance, a dish called kibbeh (kibby) in the Arab world is eaten only on happy occasions. Here in the United States we do not attach that much significance to food, and we don't have to, but it's nice to be aware of these things. Another interesting thing is that in many Middle Eastern countries yogurt and milk are never eaten with fish because of religious beliefs.

Included here are a few of the most typical recipes of the various countries. There are cookbooks available that will give you the wealth of Middle Eastern, Turkish, and Greek cooking. I have chosen the simpler and more popular recipes with which to initiate you into this new world of food.

Because you "stretch" most meat dishes by adding vegetables, they become very inexpensive and are also quite healthy. Imagine being able to trim your figure and budget at the same time? Norma F. didn't believe it was possible.

One evening I attended a small dinner party at Norma's home in the Poconos. Dinner was delicious, but it included too many carbohydrates.

After dinner, Norma confided that because of high prices she often bought too many carbohydrates since they were cheaper, and consequently she and her husband had extensive, matching midriffs. I began telling Norma about my diet plan, utilizing healthy leftovers such as vegetables and salads that would save her money in the long run.

Saving money was the key phrase, and Norma began a Middle Eastern household diet plan. She became so involved in her new way of life that she wrote and asked me to send her some exercises to firm her new figure.

One year later Norma began a small Oriental dancing school

where she teaches neighbors and friends how to live healthier and more interesting lives. She is not only saving money, but making extra money and still giving delicious but healthier dinner parties.

Not many dessert recipes have been included, and for a very good reason. Sweet "nothings" are okay when they are being whispered to you by your favorite person; however, they are too fattening in the forms of cakes and candy, and I am a firm believer, as I said before, that anything with refined sugar in it is very bad for your body. This bears repeating. If you must make yourself desserts, substitute honey for sugar. I have always thought of honey as a kind of elixir of the gods—as something good and pure. Those little bees work so hard at making this substance. They add no artificial processing to their labor of love. Have you ever looked into a jar of honey and noticed how pure and golden it appears? Wouldn't you rather have this golden substance grace your tea or whatever rather than some refined-to-death, white, powdery substance? Another good suggestion would be to substitute fresh fruit for these slurpy sweet desserts. The desserts served in the Middle East are particularly delicious, but they are also extremely fattening. If you eat any of them, make sure they do not contain sugar.

We all have a personal responsibility for our own health and well-being, and sugar does bad things to the mind and body.

Many noted nutritionists also discourage the use of sugar. About the only people who advocate the use of refined sugar are the sugar lobbyists in Washington, D.C. and the vast sugar empires. That should tell us a great deal.

You have heard of the "sweet tooth" haven't you? Well, addictive foods may not only take the form of sweets. Your addictive food may be very different from mine. For example, the most commonly addictive food substance is sweets, but many people are addicted to other substances; for example, starches such as spaghetti and bread. These are the ones I have trouble with, but I have learned to handle them very well, just as my friend Colleen Z. learned to handle her sweet tooth.

One of my friends, Colleen Z., a petite blond, always had a problem losing some marginal pounds that spoiled her appearance. She was always 5 to 8 pounds above her favorite, attractive weight because she used to get bored with dieting—and she also had a sweet tooth.

My eating pattern worked for her because it was the shock of eating a whole new group of exotic foods and getting into Oriental dancing that maintained her interest and burned off the extra calories. It took her only two weeks after she got converted to get rid of the extra 8 pounds.

I see her often these days, and her petite figure is intact. She hasn't become a professional dancer, but she is very active in the Oriental dance world, attending dance classes on a regular basis.

Her sweet tooth is completely cured, and Colleen says that she feels much better without poisonous, refined sugars in her body. If you eliminate this from your diet, you will feel better too.

It is up to you to try to control this addictive intake. If you have a difficult time, one thing you can do to help yourself is to stop buying boxes upon boxes of candies, spaghetti, or whatever your addiction may be. If you do buy them, try to buy only a limited amount. However, if they are not in the house you can't eat them, can you? Another thing you can do is to ask the members of your family, or a roommate, if you have one, to help you through the "difficult" days. They should be pretty good at reprimanding you when you reach for that extra cookie or second helping of mashed potatoes.

Even nutritious things can make you fat if you eat too much of them. I had a great problem with this. When I started to become more aware of my eating habits I used to visit health food stores and buy everything in sight. It turned out that for some reason I thought that because it was good for me I could eat unlimited amounts and I would retain my trim figure. Wrong. All of a sudden I started to gain weight. Sure enough, it finally dawned on me that I was stuffing myself silly with health foods and making myself unhealthy. This was true irony at work! I immediately cut down on my trips to the health food stores, and when I did go I bought things very carefully and sparingly.

If you are addicted to bread as my friend Lisa F. was, then you can appreciate what I am about to say. Lisa would eat four or five slices of bread with gobs of butter on them in addition to other carbo-hydrates at each meal. There is no doubt in my mind that everyone needs some bread in his or her eating pattern, but Lisa was overdoing it. I suggested to her that she try confining her bread eating to break-fast and dinner or any two of her meals for awhile. After she did that I then suggested that she buy those loaves of diet bread with the slices cut so thin you can see through them. She thought I was kidding, but I convinced her that since she had to feel as if she was eating a lot of bread, this method would help her because psychologically she would still be eating her three slices of bread, but if the bread were thin she would be outsmarting her palate and her eyes. At first it was hard for her, but I asked her brother to help her and it worked. Today she's down to two slices of whole-wheat bread per day, and she is feeling and looking a lot better for it. She is also using butter in moderation. You can do this too. Just think how much better you are going to feel if you don't stuff yourself silly. You, like Lisa F., could do without an extra 25 pounds.

If you are going around the house not knowing why you feel so sluggish, one of the reasons may be that you're eating too many carbohydrates. Just pull up the reins and slow down.

The foods of the Middle East can be fattening if you abuse them. I am going to give you a quick tour through the Middle East with my recipes. It is very hard to distinguish between the cooking of the Middle East, Turkey, and Greece. The Ottoman Turks surely left their mark all over the Arab world. Of course through the years, as with the music, dance, and other cultural features of that area, each region has developed its regional specialties. However, the more discerning palate can tell where certain dishes originated just by tasting them—the spices and oils used give the regions away.

There is a great deal of similarity between the Greek and Turkish cuisine. There is even some controversy over which dishes are Turkish and which are Greek. It is said that after the fall of Constantinople the Greeks were still under massive pressure to call their dishes by Turkish names, so even today many of the Greek dishes still have Turkish names. I am definitely not going to get into that controversy because I do not know whether this question will ever be solved. Needless to say you get a different picture from each side.

The similarity between Greek and Turkish cuisine is uncanny. I find that the Middle Eastern (Arabic) style of cooking is easier to differentiate from Greek and Turkish cuisine than to try to differentiate between the Greek and Turkish styles.

Listed here are some of the more common names that you will hear around the world of Middle Eastern, Turkish, and Greek foods. Vive le difference, or shall we say, vive the lack of difference?

Boereks are made with ready-made filo (phyllo—yufka in Turkish) pastry dough. Women in the Middle East still roll their own. You can really have fun making these: cheese boerek, chopped meat boerek, spinach boerek, and a host of others. You can make large pies or individual bite-sized delicacies. The famous spanakopitta (Greek spinach pie), well-known here in the United States, is a boerek. In Turkish it is called Ispanakli Börek.

Baklava is a great dessert of filo (strudel leaves) pastry filled with walnuts and almonds and soaked in syrup. I haven't included this in my recipes because this dessert is usually made with sugar, and this is too rich for my eating pattern, and you know how I feel about sugar. Anyway you should become familiar with the name.

Dolma is the Turkish word used to describe stuffings of all sorts of goodies into vegetables. The more popular vegetables used for dolmas are: artichokes, cabbage, eggplant, grapevine leaves, green peppers, tomatoes, and zucchini. Into these vegetables are stuffed meat and rice with all sorts of spices. Dolmas are eaten hot or cold, depending upon the kind of stuffing used. Meat dolmas are usually eaten hot, rice dolmas are eaten cold.

Kebab (Kebob) refers to cubed meats that are either baked, broiled, or stewed. Shish (şiş in Turkish) kebab, meaning "broiled meat," is the most popular form in the United States. Everyone knows shish kebab because it is served in all Greek, Middle Eastern, and Turkish restaurants, and in many American restaurants. It has been taken out of the gourmet restaurants and become very popular in the Greek souvlaki stands, so it has reached the palates of the ordinary man in the street. Kebabs are definitely more of a Turkish and Greek dish than an Arab dish.

Kibbeh (Kibby) is the national dish of Syria, Lebanon, Algeria, and many other Arab countries. It is made with bulgur (burghul) and chopped lamb or beef. Kibbeh takes all sorts of forms, sizes, and shapes. You can fry, broil, and bake it, and even eat it raw. You can roll it in balls, make it flat, or make it the shape of a football.

Kofte is the term used for meatballs.

Pastilla is a typical Moroccan dish made of pigeons and almonds wrapped in a light, delicate pastry. Pigeons are very popular in many Middle Eastern countries.

Pilav—Rice in Turkish cooking takes on a multiplicity of forms. In Turkey one never eats plain rice unless one is sick. Rice is eaten in dolmas, with peas, beans, tomatoes, pine nuts, and raisins to name a few. Rice is always cooked in some sort of stock such as chicken or lamb, but hardly ever in plain water.

Tajine is a typical Moroccan dish made of sheep mutton, almonds, and prunes.

The recipes are given English names so that you will know what you are cooking. When it is a Middle Eastern recipe I have given the Arabic, Greek, or Turkish name for that dish also. Some of the dishes have nothing to do with that part of the world; however, I have included them because they are some nutritional favorites of mine, especially the salads, and I have had a great deal of success preparing them for my friends over the years. Happy eating! And don't go back for seconds, even though you will be dying to do so.

Egg and Lemon Soup

Avgolemono—Greek   serves 6

8 cups lamb or beef stock (I like to make my stock from fresh meat bones)
½ cup rice
1½ tablespoons cornstarch
1 cup milk
3 egg yolks
¼ cup lemon juice
1 tablespoon butter
3 sprigs fresh parsley, finely chopped
salt and pepper to taste

---

1. Place stock and rice in a large saucepan and cook for about 10 minutes.
2. In a bowl mix the cornstarch, milk, and egg yolks thoroughly.
3. Add mixture to the stock very slowly and stir gently.
4. Remove from heat and add lemon juice slowly while stirring it so that it does not curdle.
5. Then before serving mix in butter and parsley.
6. Serve immediately.

The Greeks sometimes substitute very fine noodles for the rice.

Artichoke Salad

Yerelmasi Salatasi—Turkish   serves 6

2 cans artichoke hearts, drained and washed
a few large lettuce leaves
2 scallions, chopped

¼ cup fresh mint leaves, chopped
¼ cup lemon juice
¼ cup oil
3 sprigs fresh parsley, finely chopped
salt and pepper to taste
1 medium tomato, sliced (optional)

1. Cut hairy bottom off artichokes.
2. Place whole lettuce leaves at the bottom of a serving bowl.
3. Fill with artichokes.
4. Garnish top with scallions and mint leaves.
5. Pour lemon juice, oil, and parsley over artichokes and serve cold.
6. Garnish with tomato slices.

Avocado, Watercress and Shrimp Surprise   serves 6

3 large avocados
1 lb. shrimp, cooked, cleaned, and cut in cubes
1 bunch watercress, finely chopped
1 cup fresh mushrooms, sliced
½ cup water
¼ cup lime juice
½ cup cream cheese
½ cup French dressing
salt and pepper to taste

1. Steam mushrooms in water for 5 minutes and set aside to cool.
2. Cut avocados in half lengthwise and remove seeds.
3. Scoop out some of the avocado meat and leave approximately ¼" next to the skin.
4. Mix scooped-out avocado meat, lime juice, and cream cheese together.
5. Mix shrimp and watercress.
6. Place shrimp and watercress mixture in avocado shells.
7. Place cream cheese mixture on top.
8. Place mushrooms on top.
9. Pour on French dressing.
10. Refrigerate and serve cold.

Cabbage Salad

Lâhana Salatasi—Turkish   serves 4

1 medium cabbage
⅓ cup fresh parsley, chopped
1 small jar roasted red peppers, cut into strips
8 black seedless olives, chopped
¼ cup lemon juice
¼ cup oil
salt and pepper to taste

1. Cut cabbage in quarters and wash thoroughly.
2. Shred cabbage finely.
3. Place in a bowl and add salt; mix thoroughly.
4. Wash well with cold water.
5. Put in a colander and drain off all excess water.
6. Place drained cabbage in a serving bowl and add parsley, peppers, olives, lemon juice, and oil.
7. Serve cold.

Cauliflower Salad

Karnibahar Salatasi—Turkish   serves 8

1 medium cauliflower, washed and cleaned
1 quart water
2 tablespoons lemon juice
3 hard-boiled eggs, sliced thin
6 black olives
5 radishes, sliced fine
2 scallions, finely chopped
2 tablespoons fresh parsley, chopped
salt and pepper to taste

1. Bring water to boil in a saucepan, add lemon juice, salt and pepper.
2. Add the whole cauliflower, steam until tender (approximately 15 minutes), allow to cool.

3. Cut cauliflower and arrange in salad bowl.
4. Arrange eggs around cauliflower.
5. Garnish with olives, radishes, scallions, and parsley.
6. Serve cold.

Chef's Salad   serves 8

2 cups salad greens, cleaned
1 cucumber, sliced
2 carrots, cleaned and sliced
1 can artichoke hearts, drained and sliced
1 small tomato, cubed
3 scallions, finely chopped
3 ounces low-fat cheese, cut in strips
2 cups cold lean meat, cut in strips
1 tablespoon lemon juice
1 tablespoon oil
salt and pepper to taste

---

1. Mix all the ingredients together.
2. Serve cold.

Chicken Vegetable Salad   serves 8

2 cups white meat of chicken or turkey, chopped
½ cup celery, peeled and diced
½ cup water chestnuts, drained and sliced
¼ cup green pepper, diced
¼ cup pimento, chopped
¼ cup scallions, sliced
¼ cup mayonnaise
salt and pepper to taste

---

1. Mix all ingredients together.
2. Serve cold.

Dried Bean Salad

Piyaz—Turkish   serves 6

1 can white kidney or navy beans
3 tablespoons oil
1½ tablespoons lemon juice
2 scallions, finely chopped
1 teaspoon fresh dill (½ teaspoon if dried)
1 hard boiled egg, sliced
4 sprigs fresh parsley, chopped
12 black olives
salt and pepper to taste

1. Drain beans and place in a serving dish.
2. Add oil, lemon juice, scallions, salt and pepper and mix thoroughly but gently.
3. Garnish with eggs, parsley and olives.
4. Refrigerate and serve cold.

Eggplant Salad

Patlican Salatasi—Turkish
Salata il Batinjan—Arabic   serves 4

5 medium eggplants
¼ cup oil
¼ cup lemon juice
1 teaspoon wine vinegar
½ teaspoon garlic powder
1 green pepper, sliced in strips
1 large tomato, sliced thin
1 onion, sliced thin
8 black olives
salt and pepper to taste

1. Place the whole eggplants on foil paper or a roasting pan in the oven (about 400°).
2. Cook until skin turns black and begins to shrivel; make sure to turn eggplants occasionally so that all sides cook.
3. Take skin off when eggplant is still hot (skin will come off easily).

4. Place eggplant in a bowl.
5. Add oil, lemon, vinegar, and garlic powder and mash mixture thoroughly until smooth.
6. Place in a salad plate and garnish with pepper, tomato, onion, and olives.
7. Serve cold.
8. May be eaten with pita bread.

Greek Salad   serves 6

1 head lettuce, washed and chopped
3 large tomatoes, cut in eighths
1 large cucumber, sliced
1 onion, sliced lengthwise
1 green pepper, chopped
½ cup oil
¼ cup vinegar
1 small can, or ¼ lb., Greek olives, black
1 can fillets of anchovies
½ lb. feta cheese, sliced into ¼" slabs
salt and pepper to taste

1. Mix all ingredients except olives, anchovies, and cheese together in a large salad bowl.
2. Garnish with olives, anchovies, and feta cheese.

Romaine Lettuce Salad

Marul Salatasi—Turkish   serves 6

1 romaine lettuce
3 scallions, chopped
¼ cup fresh mint leaves, chopped
¼ cup lemon juice
¼ cup oil
¼ teaspoon garlic powder
3 tablespoons fresh parsley, chopped
salt and pepper to taste

1. Wash and clean the lettuce well.
2. Tear the lettuce leaves into small pieces with your hands and put in a salad bowl.
3. Garnish with scallions and mint leaves.
4. Mix lemon juice, oil, and garlic together and pour over lettuce; add parsley.

Note: Lettuce leaves should never be cut with a knife—you injure them! The edges will turn brown if you have to refrigerate them.

Shepherd's Salad
Çoban Salatasi—Turkish   serves 8

1 medium onion, sliced vertically
1 cup cold water
1 tablespoon salt
½ head romaine lettuce, shredded
1 cucumber, sliced thin
1 large tomato, sliced thin
3 radishes, sliced
1 green pepper, sliced thin
1 small jar roasted red peppers, finely chopped
8 black olives
2 scallions, finely chopped
2 tablespoons fresh parsley, chopped
2 tablespoons fresh dill, chopped
2 tablespoons fresh mint leaves, chopped
½ cup lemon juice
¼ cup oil
1 teaspoon wine vinegar
1 teaspoon garlic powder
salt and pepper to taste

1. Place sliced onion, water, and salt in a bowl and knead onion thoroughly, then drain off water and place onion in salad bowl.
2. Place all ingredients in a mixing bowl and mix thoroughly together.
3. Place in a salad bowl.
4. Serve cold.

Spinach Salad

Ispanakli Salatasi—Turkish   serves 4

2 pounds fresh spinach
2 cups water
salt and pepper to taste
1 medium onion, sliced vertically
2 cups cold water
1 tablespoon salt
¼ cup oil
juice of 2 lemons (¼ cup)
1 teaspoon wine vinegar
2 hard-boiled eggs, sliced thin
10 black olives

---

1. Place spinach in water, bring to a boil, and steam about 5 minutes; drain.
2. Place sliced onion, 1 cup water, and salt in a bowl and knead onion thoroughly, then drain off water, wash with balance of water, drain, and place onion in salad bowl.
3. Place oil, lemon juice, and vinegar in bowl, adding salt and pepper; mix thoroughly.
4. Put thoroughly drained spinach in the salad bowl.
5. Pour lemon and oil sauce over the spinach and onion; mix thoroughly.
6. Place sliced eggs on the top.
7. Garnish with olives.

Tomato and Cucumber Salad

Domates Ve Hiyr Salatasi—Turkish   serves 4

1 cucumber, sliced lengthwise and cut in cubes
2 medium tomatoes, cut in eighths
½ tablespoon fresh mint, finely chopped
1 tablespoon fresh dill, finely chopped
1 scallion, chopped
2 tablespoons oil
1 tablespoon lemon juice
1 teaspoon wine vinegar
salt and pepper to taste

1. Arrange cucumber and tomatoes on a flat platter.
2. Garnish with mint, dill, and scallion.
3. Pour oil, lemon juice, and vinegar over salad.
4. Serve cold.

Tomato and Onion Salad

Sovanli Domates Salatasi—Turkish   serves 4

2 medium onions
2 cups cold water
2 large tomatoes
1 can fillets of anchovies
2 tablespoons fresh parsley, chopped
¼ cup oil
¼ cup lemon juice
salt and pepper to taste

1. Place sliced onion, 1 cup water, and salt in a bowl and knead onion thoroughly, then drain off water.
2. Wash with balance of water and drain again.
3. Wash tomatoes and cut into eighths.
4. Put tomatoes and onions on a plate.
5. Garnish with fillets of anchovies and parsley.
6. Pour oil and lemon juice over salad.

Zucchini Salad

Kabak Salatasi—Turkish   serves 8

5 medium zucchini
1 cup water
1 teaspoon salt
2 large tomatoes, cut in wedges
3 hard-boiled eggs, sliced in ¼" slices
1 medium onion
2 cups cold water
1 tablespoon salt

1 medium green pepper, finely chopped
2 scallions, chopped
2 tablespoons fresh dill
12 black olives
2 tablespoons fresh parsley, chopped
½ cup lemon juice
½ cup oil
pepper to taste

---

1. Wash and cut zucchini into ½" slices
2. Steam zucchini in water, which has been salted, until tender, approximately 5 minutes.
3. Cool and drain.
4. Arrange on a flat plate.
5. Add tomato wedges and egg slices.
6. Place sliced onion, 1 cup water, and salt in a bowl and knead onion thoroughly, then drain off water.
7. Wash with balance of water and drain again.
8. Place over zucchini.
9. Place green pepper, scallions, and dill over zucchini.
10. Garnish with olives and parsley.
11. Pour lemon juice and oil over salad.

Onion Eggs, Scrambled

Sovanli Yumurta—Turkish　　　　　　serves 4

4 onions, finely sliced
2 tablespoons oil
4 eggs
⅛ teaspoon allspice
salt and pepper to taste

---

1. Sauté onions in oil in frying pan until golden brown.
2. Whip eggs in mixing bowl with salt, pepper, and allspice.
3. Pour mixture on top of onions and scramble until eggs are done.
4. Serve immediately.

Onion Eggs, Fried
Sovanli Yumurta

1. Sauté onions in oil in frying pan until golden brown.
2. Break eggs, one at a time, on top of bed of onions.
3. Sprinkle with salt, pepper, and allspice.
4. Cover and cook until eggs are done.
5. Serve immediately.

Spinach Eggs

Ispanakli Yumurta—Turkish   serves 4

1 package frozen chopped spinach or 2 bags fresh spinach, cooked
2 tablespoons polyunsaturated margarine
1 large onion, finely chopped
1 teaspoon honey
½ teaspoon paprika
½ cup grated parmesan cheese
4 eggs
salt and pepper to taste

1. Sauté onion in margarine in a frying pan until golden brown.
2. Add cooked spinach and stir frequently for about 5 minutes.
3. Add honey, salt, and pepper and blend everything together well; let simmer a few minutes.
4. Sprinkle parmesan cheese on top of mixture.
5. Break eggs on top of the bed of spinach.
6. Sprinkle with paprika.
7. Cover and cook until eggs are done to your liking.
8. Serve immediately.

Carrot Plaki

Havuç Plakisi—Turkish   serves 6

8 medium carrots, washed, scraped and cut in ½ circles
2 cups water

2 large onions, cut in diagonal strips
¼ cup oil
1 tablespoon rice
2 tablespoons lemon juice
1 teaspoon honey
1 lemon cut in wedges
6 springs parsley, chopped
salt and pepper to taste

1. Sauté onions in oil until golden brown in a large saucepan.
2. Add carrots and water to saucepan and steam about 10 minutes.
3. Add rice, lemon juice, honey, and salt and pepper.
4. Continue to cook until most of the water has evaporated and carrots are tender.
5. Place mixture in serving dish and allow to cool.
6. Garnish with parsley and lemon wedges.
7. Serve cold.

Green Beans with Oil

Zeytinyagli Fasulye—Turkish
Fasoulakia Yahni—Greek   serves 6

1 lb. fresh string beans, washed and cut French style
1 cup water
3 tablespoons oil
1 tablespoon lemon juice
1 medium onion
2 large tomatoes, chopped, or 1 16 oz. can peeled tomatoes
1 medium green pepper, finely chopped
½ teaspoon thyme
1 clove garlic, finely chopped
½ teaspoon honey
salt and pepper to taste

1. Place all ingredients in a saucepan and steam over a low flame until beans are tender (about ½ hour).
2. Remove from heat and allow to cool.
3. Serve cold.

Couscous—Moroccan   serves 8

This is usually made in a special pot called a couscoussiere; however, you can use a colander that will fit tightly into a saucepan.

2 cups couscous
2 quarts water
1 lb. lamb, cut into 2" cubes
3 large onions, chopped
1 tablespoon turmeric
¼ teaspoon cayenne pepper
2 sprigs fresh parsley, finely chopped
1 tablespoon ground ginger
½ cup oil
10 tablespoons butter
¼ teaspoon saffron, crushed
2 medium turnips
4 medium carrots, washed, peeled, and cut into 4 pieces
1 large potato, washed, peeled, and cut into 8 pieces
2 zucchini, washed, cut into 1" pieces with skin left on
1 can chickpeas (1 lb., 4 oz.)
1 cup seedless raisins or currants
salt and pepper to taste

1. Place couscous in large saucepan and add enough water (about 1 qt.) to just about cover it.
2. Let sit for about one hour, occasionally mixing with your hand to avoid lumpiness.
3. Soak saffron in a little warm water.
4. Place lamb, onions, turmeric, cayenne pepper, parsley, ginger, ¼ cup of oil, six tablespoons of butter, saffron, and salt and pepper in the bottom part of the couscoussiere (in the saucepan if you do not have a couscoussiere); add balance of water and boil over low flame (about 15 minutes).
5. Place steamer part of couscoussiere (colander if that is being used) on top of couscoussiere bottom.
6. Line steamer (colander) with cheesecloth and add couscous.
7. Cover and cook over medium flame for about ½ hour.
8. Remove steamer (colander) and run cold water over couscous; drain and mix with your hands to get out any lumps.
9. Set couscous aside to drain.
10. Add turnips, carrots, and potato to bottom of couscoussiere (saucepan) and cook for 15 minutes.
11. Place couscous in a large bowl, add ¼ cup oil and salt to taste, and mix thoroughly with your hands (a wooden spoon would be fine if you are squeamish).

12. Add zucchini, chickpeas and raisins to stew.
13. Replace steamer (colander) on top with couscous and continue to cook for 10 more minutes.
14. Add remaining butter to couscous and place in a large serving dish.
15. Make a well in the center and place lamb and vegetables in it.
16. Serve hot.

Gardener's Kebab

Bahçivan Kebabi—Turkish   serves 4

1½ lbs. lamb, cut in 1" cubes
2 cups water
3 tablespoons oil
3 large carrots, peeled and sliced in ½" circles
3 medium tomatoes
1½ lbs. pearl onions
1 cup fresh green peas
salt and pepper to taste
½ teaspoon thyme
¼ teaspoon cumin
1 teaspoon fresh dill (½ teaspoon if dried)

1. Brown meat in oil in a saucepan.
2. Add water.
3. Cook covered over low flame for about ½ hour.
4. Add carrots, tomatoes, onions, peas, thyme, cumin, salt and pepper.
5. Stir occasionally.
6. Add dill shortly before serving.

Spinach Pie

Spanakopitta—Greek
Ispanakli Boerek—Turkish   serves 8

4 large onions, chopped
1 bunch scallions, finely chopped
1 cup oil

1 bunch fresh parsley, finely chopped
3 lbs. fresh spinach
½ cup fresh dill, finely chopped
1 lb. feta cheese, chopped in chunks
1 box filo (phyllo) pastry
salt and pepper to taste

1. Brown onions and scallions in oil in a saucepan and remove from fire.
2. Wash spinach thoroughly and finely chop; discard bottom stems and add to onions.
3. Add parsley, dill, cheese, salt and pepper.
4. Stir thoroughly.
5. Take a baking pan and grease lightly.
6. Line bottom and sides with about 6 filo leaves.
7. Spread evenly half of the spinach mixture over the filo leaves.
8. Cover with a couple of filo leaves, leaving some to cover the top.
9. Place remaining spinach mixture on top of filo.
10. Cover top with remaining filo leaves, tucking the ends in neatly.
11. Brush the top with oil and stick little holes with a fork.
12. Bake in oven (350°) for about ½ hour (filo leaves should be golden brown).

You can make little boereks with this mixture by taking filo leaves and cutting them in small pieces, then adding about a teaspoon of the spinach mixture and wrapping and folding the filo around it to form a cigarette-shaped boerek. Place on a greased baking dish and bake for about 15 minutes.

Vegetable Pot

Türlü—Turkish   serves 6

1 lb. lamb, cut into 1″ cubes
2 large onions
¼ cup oil
2 cups water
¼ teaspoon thyme
½ teaspoon cumin
salt and pepper to taste

½ lb. fresh string beans, cut French style
2 zucchini, cut into 1″ slices
½ lb. fresh okra
2 large green peppers, chopped
1 large potato, cubed
2 large tomatoes, chopped
2 small eggplants, cut into 1″ cubes, leaving skin on

_____

1. Brown onions in a large saucepan.
2. Add meat, thyme, cumin, salt and pepper and continue to brown.
3. Add 1 cup of water and simmer for about 15 minutes.
4. Add all vegetables.
5. Add other cup of water.
6. Cook for about 15 minutes until vegetables are done.
7. Serve hot.

In Turkey they vary this for the summer (Yaz) and winter (Kis) depending on what vegetables are available. This recipe is the summer version.

Baked Kibby

Kibbeh—Arabic   serves 8

Basic Kibby
1 lb. lean lamb, ground three or four times
1 large onion, grated
2 cups burghul, fine
salt and freshly ground black pepper

_____

1. Combine lamb and onion and mix thoroughly with hands, in a mortar pounded with a pestle if you have one.
2. Wash the burghul in a colander lined with cheesecloth under running water, but do it quickly so burghul does not soften.
3. Combine lamb and burghul with salt and pepper and mix thoroughly, kneading with your hands until it has a pasty consistency.
4. Set aside and make stuffing.

Stuffing
½ lb. lamb, ground twice

1 cup chopped onion
½ cup pine nuts
⅓ cup oil
¼ teaspoon cinnamon
salt and pepper to taste

---

1. Heat oil and sauté onion until soft.
2. Add meat and sauté until lightly browned.
3. Add pine nuts and sauté until they are lightly browned and meat has lost all pink color.
4. Season with salt, pepper, and cinnamon.
5. Pour off all excess oil.

Assembling the kibby

¾ cup clarified butter (samneh in Arabic)
This is made by melting butter in a warm oven and straining it through fine muslin. One cup of butter will make ¾ cup of clarified butter.

---

1. Grease a shallow pan, approximately 12″ x 14″.
2. Take a little less than half of the basic kibby and pat it over the pan.
3. Smooth the stuffing evenly over the bottom layer.
4. Pat the remaining basic kibby over the stuffing.
5. Score through the three layers with a sharp knife, making a diamond pattern.
6. Pour the clarified butter over the top.
7. Bake in a moderate oven (375°) about 20 minutes, or until it is well browned.
8. Serve hot.

Meat and Okra

Etli Bamya—Turkish   serves 6

1½ lbs. lamb or beef, ground
2 boxes frozen whole okra, or 18 fresh okra parboiled
1 large onion, chopped
2 tablespoons oil

1 16 oz. can peeled tomatoes or 2 large tomatoes, chopped
½ teaspoon thyme
2 tablespoons lemon juice
salt and pepper to taste
2 cups water

1. Sauté onions in oil until golden brown.
2. Add meat and sauté for a few minutes until brown.
3. Add tomatoes and 1 cup water; cook for 10 minutes more.
4. Add okra, salt, pepper, thyme, lemon juice, and balance of water.
5. Cover and cook slowly for about ½ hour until most of the water is gone.

Meat Balls Kebab

Kôfte Kebab or Şiş Kôfte—Turkish
Mow-a-seer—Arabic   serves 6

2 lbs. ground round steak or mutton
1 large onion, finely chopped
1 teaspoon paprika
1 teaspoon oregano
¼ teaspoon cumin
2 eggs
½ cup seasoned bread crumbs
salt and pepper to taste
1 tablespoon oil
6 skewers

1. Mix all ingredients together and marinate for about ½ hour.
2. Shape into 4" or 5" rolls and string them on a skewer.
3. Broil for a few minutes over a charcoal grill or in the oven broiler.

You can add slices of onions, green peppers, mushrooms, and tomatoes between the meat for variety.

Raw Beef—Steak Tartare

Lahum Nee—Syrian   serves 2

½ lb. ground meat, top quality beef fillet, sirloin or round steak
1 large onion, finely chopped
¼ teaspoon thyme
salt and pepper to taste

1. Knead ingredients together.
2. Make into flat patties and serve.

This is especially good for the tigers in your family!

Lamb Brains

Beyin Haşlamasi—Turkish   serves 4

4 lamb brains
3 cups water
salt to taste
¼ cup lemon juice (juice of 2 lemons)
2 tablespoons oil
2 sprigs fresh parsley, finely chopped
a few lettuce leaves

1. Boil brains in water for about 10 minutes.
2. Add salt.
3. Drain water and leave brains to cool.
4. Cut brains into small flat pieces and place on a flat bed of lettuce.
5. Cover with lemon juice, oil, and garnish with parsley.
6. Serve cold.

Veal Cutlet with Zucchini   serves 4

4 veal cutlets
2 egg whites, beaten

½ cup bread crumbs
1 tablespoon oil
1 cup canned tomatoes
⅛ teaspoon oregano
⅛ teaspoon thyme
2 medium zucchini, sliced ½" thick
salt and pepper to taste

---

1. Dip cutlets in egg whites, then in crumbs.
2. Brown them in oil.
3. Pour off excess oil, add tomatoes, salt, pepper, oregano, thyme; cover and simmer 30 minutes.
4. Add zucchini and continue cooking for approximately 30 minutes.

Other vegetables may be used instead of zucchini.

The Imam Fainted

Patlican Imambayildi—Turkish   serves 4

2 large eggplants
1 cup oil
3 large onions, finely chopped
3 large tomatoes, 2 finely chopped, 1 sliced in thin slices
½ lb. ground meat (lamb or beef)
1 clove garlic, finely chopped, or 1 teaspoon garlic powder
1 bunch parsley, finely chopped
salt and pepper to taste
1 cup meat stock
½ teaspoon thyme
¼ teaspoon cumin

---

1. Peel skin of eggplants in strips so that you have alternate strips of purple and white.
2. Cut eggplants in half lengthwise and place in a casserole or baking pan.
3. Place in oven until tops of eggplants are lightly brown.
4. Remove from oven and scoop out some of the seeds in the middle so that a little well is formed.
5. In a frying pan brown onions in oil.
6. Add chopped tomatoes and continue to brown.

7. Add salt, pepper, thyme, and cumin.
8. Add chopped meat and stir until brown.
9. Place meat mixture on top of eggplants.
10. Garnish with tomato slices and parsley.
11. Add meat stock around eggplants.
12. Return casserole to oven (350°) and bake for about 15 more minutes.
13. Serve hot.

Hawaiian Chicken a la Linda

1 chicken, quartered
1 bottle French dressing
1 jar apricot preserves, natural—no sugar added
½ package dry onion soup mix
2 tablespoons polyunsaturated margarine

---

1. Mix all the ingredients and marinate overnight.
2. Arrange in a pan and bake in a 450° oven until golden brown, approximately 1½ hours.

This dish is dedicated to my good friend Linda. Linda is not what you would call your basic gourmet cook; in fact she found out where the kitchen was very late in life. However, at least once a year she comes up with a beauty. It's always an easy dish to prepare, but it looks as if you've slaved for hours over it.

Roast Chicken with Pine Nut and Currant Stuffing
Piliç Dolmasi—Turkish   serves 6

1 roasting chicken
4 medium potatoes
2 lemons, cut in halves
1 large onion, finely chopped
1 bunch scallions, finely chopped (use only white part)
2 tablespoons polyunsaturated margarine
¼ cup pine nuts
1 tablespoon parsley, chopped

1 teaspoon garlic powder
1 teaspoon thyme
1½ quarts water
3 tablespoons tomato paste
salt and pepper to taste

---

1. Wash chicken thoroughly with lemons.
2. Cook potatoes for 15 minutes; mash and set aside.
3. Sauté onion and scallions in margarine, add nuts, currants, garlic, and parsley; sauté a few minutes longer until the nuts are slightly brown.
4. Add mashed potatoes; mix all ingredients together and set aside to cool.
5. Fill chicken with this stuffing and sew up bottom and neck of the chicken.
6. Place chicken in roasting pan, add water, tomato paste, salt, pepper, and thyme.
7. Roast for about 1½ hours in a 350° oven; baste every 20 minutes.

Baked Bluefish   serves 4

1 3 lb. bluefish, cleaned, bones removed, split lengthwise
5 strips bacon, cut in halves
¼ cup fresh parsley, chopped
1 tablespoon dill, chopped
1 medium onion, finely chopped
1 lemon, cut in wedges
salt and pepper to taste
1½ cups sour cream

---

1. Preheat oven to 400°.
2. Put fish, skin side down, in greased baking pan.
3. Put bacon strips over fish.
4. Add dill and onion.
5. Bake approximately 20 minutes.
6. Remove from oven, cover with sour cream, and top with parsley.
7. Serve hot.

Porgies (Broiled)   serves 4

2 porgies
salt and pepper to taste
¼ cup butter, melted
¼ cup flour
1 teaspoon paprika
¼ teaspoon thyme

1. Add salt and pepper to porgies.
2. Pour half of butter over porgies.
3. Sprinkle half the flour on fish.
4. Place in broiling pan and broil for 10 minutes.
5. Turn and pour on rest of butter.
6. Sprinkle on rest of flour, paprika and thyme.
7. Broil until fish is flaky, approximately 10 minutes.

Swordfish Kebab

Kiliç Şişte—Turkish
Souvlakia—Greek   serves 4

3 lbs. swordfish
2 tablespoons lemon juice
2 tablespoons oil
1 tablespoon onion juice
1 teaspoon thyme
½ tablespoon paprika
¼ teaspoon oregano
salt and pepper to taste
1 dozen bay leaves
4 skewers

1. Skin and cut the fish into 1" cubes.
2. Marinate fish in mixture of lemon juice, oil, onion juice,
   thyme, paprika, oregano, salt and pepper for several hours in
   the refrigerator.
3. Place fish on skewers, placing a bay leaf between cubes.
4. Broil over charcoal or in oven broiler until cooked.

You can also make this like a meat kebab by placing various vegetables like tomatoes or onions between fish cubes.

Dolmas—Stuffed Vegetables

Turkish and Greek   serves 8

1½ lbs. ground lamb or beef
2 onions, finely chopped
½ cup unprocessed rice
1 teaspoon fresh mint, chopped
1 teaspoon fresh dill, chopped
1 teaspoon cumin
¼ cup tomato sauce
¼ cup parsley, chopped
8 large tomatoes (you can substitute green peppers, squash, or a small eggplant)
3 tablespoons butter
2 cups water

1. Place all ingredients except tomato sauce, tomatoes, butter, and water in a mixing bowl and knead them well with your hands.
2. Cut off the tops of tomatoes and keep them for a cover; scoop out the seeds, leaving about a ¼″ shell.
3. Stuff mixture into the shells, cover with stem end, and fasten with toothpicks.
4. Place in a saucepan.
5. Add water, tomato sauce, and butter.
6. Boil over a low flame until most of the water has evaporated, about ¾ hour.

Stuffed Grape Leaves

Warak inib mihshec—Arabic
Yalanci Dolma—Turkish
Yalandji Dolma—Greek   serves 8

4 cups water
2 16 oz. jars. of grape leaves (about 50 leaves)
3 large onions, finely chopped
2 cups unbleached rice
3 tablespoons black currants

2 tablespoons pine (pignolia) nuts
¼ cup fresh mint leaves, chopped
¼ cup fresh parsley, chopped
¼ cup fresh dill, chopped
2 tablespoons lemon juice
½ cup oil
1 teaspoon honey
1 tablespoon allspice
1 teaspoon thyme
salt and pepper to taste
lamb bones or chicken wings
2 lemons, cut in wedges

---

1. Wash and dry grape leaves and separate them as best you can without breaking them.
2. Remove tops of stems from grape leaves.
3. Fry onions in deep saucepan in oil until golden brown.
4. Add rice, currants, nuts, mint, parsley, dill, lemon juice, and honey.
5. Add 1 cup water and simmer for about 15 minutes.
6. Set aside to cool.
7. Put a grape leaf, rough side up, on a flat surface (if they are small, overlap 2 grape leaves) and place about one teaspoon of the meat mixture on the stem end of the leaf, fold stem end over, and then fold both sides toward center like an envelope and roll to end of leaf.
8. Place bones at bottom of a deep saucepan and then cover them with a few grape leaves.
9. Put filled grape leaves in the saucepan in layers; crisscross them in a sort of lattice pattern.
10. Put in balance of water, cover with wax paper, and place a plate over the wax paper to keep grape leaves from coming loose while cooking.
11. Cover with pot cover and cook over medium fire until rice is cooked and most of the water is absorbed, about ¾ hour.
12. Remove from heat; let stand until cool.
13. Carefully take out grape leaf dolmas and arrange them on a platter.
14. Garnish with lemon wedges, which you can use to squeeze on your dolmas to add more lemon.
15. Serve cold.

For variety, use cabbage leaves instead of grape leaves.

Eggplant "Pizzas"   serves 8

2 medium eggplants
2 eggs, beaten
½ box Italian-style bread crumbs
1 small jar spaghetti sauce flavored with meat
1 5 oz. pack fresh parmesan cheese, grated
oil

1. Peel eggplants and cut into ¼" slices; salt slices and let rest for several minutes until beads of water appear; dry slices with paper towels.
2. Dip eggplant into eggs; shake off excess egg and cover eggplant with bread crumbs.
3. Fry in oil until golden brown; place fried slices on paper towels to soak up excess oil.
4. Put a teaspoon of spaghetti sauce on each eggplant slice.
5. Sprinkle grated parmesan cheese on top of sauce.
6. Remove from paper towel and place on serving dish.
7. Serve warm or cold as you wish.

This is one of the few recipes I've included using fried foods. It's something different, and one can make a whole meal of it. Make this one of the "treats" you give yourself from time to time. It's also an easy dish to make for unexpected company.

Eggplant Surprise   serves 8

2 medium eggplants
oil
¼ oz. cottage cheese
½ oz. sour cream

1. Peel eggplants and cut into ¼" slices.
2. Salt slices and let rest for several minutes until beads òf water appear; dry slices with paper towels.

3. Fry slices in oil until golden brown; place fried slices on paper towels to soak up excess oil.
4. Place slices on flat dish; allow to cool.
5. When cooled, cover with cottage cheese and sour cream.

For added spice, slice 2 green peppers, fry them, and add them to the eggplant. An alternative to the cottage cheese and sour cream is a container of yogurt.

Fish-Roe Mix

Tarama—Turkish and Greek   **yields about 1½ cups**

1 jar tarama (carp roe), scales and membranes removed
¼ cup sour cream
¼ cup bread crumbs
¼ cup lemon juice
¼ cup oil
a few large lettuce leaves
8 black olives
1 sprig fresh parsley, finely chopped
1 small grated onion (optional)

---

1. Mix tarama, sour cream, and bread crumbs together with a handmixer or blender until a paste is formed.
2. Pour in lemon juice, oil slowly, and continue mixing.
3. Place lettuce leaves on a flat platter.
4. Place paste on top of lettuce leaves.
5. Garnish with olives and parsley.
6. You may also add a small grated onion if you wish.

Chick-pea Dip

Nohut Ezmesi—Turkish
Hummus bi Tahini—Arabic   **yields 1½ cups**

1 can chick-peas, drained
3 tablespoons tahini (sesame paste)

2 tablespoons oil
juice of 3 lemons, approximately ½ cup lemon juice
1 teaspoon paprika
3 tablespoons pomegranate seeds (optional)
3 tablespoons fresh parsley, chopped

1. Drain water from chickpeas and mix with a handmixer or in a blender.
2. Add tahini, lemon juice, and oil.
3. Mix all ingredients well until they turn into a paste.
4. Place in a serving dish, garnish with paprika, parsley, and pomegranate seeds.
5. Serve with flat Arabic bread (pita).

The Arabic bread is used as a sort of spoon, or if you will, as your regular cocktail cracker. In other words, don't be afraid to break off a piece of bread and dip it right into the hummus!

Eggplant Dip

Patlican Salatasi—Turkish
Baba Ghannouj—Arabic   yields 2 cups

4 large eggplants
4 tablespoons tahini (sesame paste)
½ cup lemon juice
1 tablespoon garlic powder
3 tablespoons fresh parsley, chopped
8 black olives
3 tablespoons pomegranate seeds (optional)
1 teaspoon paprika
salt to taste

1. Place foil paper on the bottom of the broiler.
2. Stick eggplants with a fork in several places; place them in the broiler and broil with the skin on, making sure to turn them frequently so that they don't stick to the foil paper.
3. Broil for about 1½ hours or until cooked inside.
4. Remove skin under cold water and mash eggplant thoroughly.
5. Add garlic powder, oil, tahini, and lemon juice.
6. Place on a flat platter and garnish with parsley, olives, pome-

granate seeds and paprika (You could also garnish with pine nuts if you wish).

7. Serve with flat Arabic bread (pita).

Avocado Dip

Taratoov Avocado—Arabic   yields 2 cups

2 avocados
3 tablespoons tahini (sesame paste)
2 tablespoons lemon juice
1 tablespoon oil
salt to taste

---

1. Cut avocado in quarters and remove seed.
2. Scoop out meat of avocado and mash it.
3. Add tahini, lemon juice, oil, and salt.
4. Mix until it becomes a paste.
5. Serve with flat Arabic bread (pita).

Ambrosia Dessert à la Joan   serves 8

1 can (3½ oz.) mandarin oranges, drained; no sugar added
1 can (15½ oz.) pineapple chunks, drained; no sugar added
5 ⅓ oz. miniature marshmallows
1 cup sour cream
2 cups fresh strawberries
1 can (3 oz.) shredded coconut
½ cup honey

---

1. Mix and marinate the mandarin oranges, pineapple chunks, marshmallows, and sour cream overnight in refrigerator.
2. Next day, add strawberries and shredded coconut; mix all ingredients together.
3. Refrigerate until ready to serve.

Another one of my dear friends' creations. Unlike Linda, Joan knows where the kitchen is. This is one of her easy ones. It is a finger-licking dessert guaranteed to please. You must promise me to eat only a small portion of this because you'll be tempted to go back for seconds, and that's no good for the waistline.

Honeyed Melon   serves 2

1 honeydew melon
1 8 oz. container sour cream
1 8 oz. container cottage cheese
2 teaspoons honey

1. Cut the melon in half; scoop out seeds and strings.
2. Fill hole with scoop of cottage cheese.
3. Add sour cream.
4. Top with honey.

For a once-in-a-while treat add some dates or finely chopped figs.

Lemon Jelly Mold à la Lebwa   serves 6

1 pack (6 oz.) lemon-flavored gelatin
2 cups boiling water
1½ cups orange juice
1 cup dates or figs, finely chopped
1 cup fresh peaches, cubed

1. Dissolve gelatin in boiling water.
2. Add orange juice and dates or figs.
3. Pour into a ring mold; approximately 1 quart will do.
4. Chill until firm.
5. Unmold and fill center of ring with fresh peaches.

Turkish Coffee

To make one cup
1 heaping teaspoon Turkish coffee
1 demitasse cup cold water
⅛ teaspoon orange blossom essence (optional)
special Turkish coffee pot called a jezve

---

1. Put cold water in jezve.
2. Add coffee and stir three times.
3. Place over flame and boil until foam starts to rise to the top of the pot. (You really have to watch this carefully so that it does not boil over.)
4. Remove pot from fire and skim off foam and put it in the coffee cup.
5. Return pot to the fire and boil once more just for a few seconds until you see the foam rising again.
6. Pour into cup and serve.
7. Add orange blossom essence to taste.

Coffee is an integral part of Middle Eastern hospitality. It is a sign of welcome. Tea sometimes acts as a respectable substitute, and anywhere you go in the Middle East, even when shopping, you'll be invited to have a cup of one or the other. Turkish coffee cannot be reheated; it has to be made fresh and served immediately.

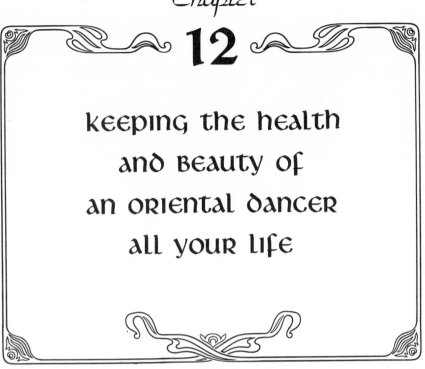

keeping the health and Beauty of an oriental dancer all your life

Somewhere in the back of my mind I have this fantasy of an Egyptian Oriental dancer of great beauty. I often picture her and try to put her together from my experiences. I have great fun doing this in museums, where I go to visit the Egyptian collections every chance I get. I recently had the good fortune to dream at the actual sites in Egypt where the Pharaohs and their queens once stood. I thought of the Pharaohs and their queens and all the splendor that must have surrounded them, and I dreamed, and dreamed, and dreamed.

Thanks to the information we have been able to salvage from Egyptian wall paintings and from archaeological digs, we can piece together a few glimpses back into that ancient culture that must have been the epitome of exoticism. I visit museums quite often, and oftentimes I wander over to the Egyptian collection, where I allow the quiet mood of intuitive concentration to help me realize this vision. On a recent vacation I visited the Egyptian museum in Cairo, where you could stay for hours and visualize a great ancient civilization. This museum is so vast you would need weeks to see it thoroughly. I never think of the Oriental dancer with the hootchy-kootchy idea that so many people hold of her.

Today, when someone calls me an exotic dancer I literally go berserk because that term has been linked with strippers for such a long time, and I don't like the association. I like to think of exotic as being something or someone of an unusual quality of beauty or an excitingly strange appearance that is hardly describable. I think of exoticism as untouchable and enchanting beauty. I think of the days of the Pharaohs and their beautiful Queens. I think of the lovely women being bathed in oils, then dressed in colorful silk gowns, and fanned with giant fans by their countless ladies-in-waiting as they sit on soft cushions with their hair flowing in the breeze, watching the dancing girls entertain them. The movie producers have helped us to go back in time and see how it may have been. Then my bubble bursts when I think of a strip joint and some emcee introducing one of his protégés as the exotic, "striptotic" beauty queen, titanic, or whatever. Oh, how I yearn for the truly *exotic* days associated with the nobility of ancient Egypt, of the Pashas of Turkey, and the beauty of the Greek temples!

As I said before, dancing in Egypt was performed mostly at ceremonial functions. Dances were also performed at royal functions, at marriages, and even at funerals. They were also performed in honor of the gods. With all this in mind, I think of the dancer as an important part of the world of being. I think of her as someone who should be pampered. If the dancer is a man then he should be pampered too. Indeed, all people should pamper their bodies to keep them in shape. You too should be pampered even though you are not on the stage—but remember, "all the world's a stage."

The ideas that I have put forth throughout this book are not ideas that you should file away for future reference. You should not start to put them into effect today and forget about them tomorrow. They are ideas that you should entertain in your mind for the rest of your life. After all, your body is going to be around that long too, and you don't want it falling apart by the wayside, do you? They are ideas that should help you gain new perspectives about your life and the course you want it to take.

Once you have achieved your goal of the desired weight for a person your age, sex, bodily structure, and chemical composition, you must be careful to maintain your weight and not let it slip back into the rut from which you dug it out. The ultimate goal in your life should be to follow a lifelong program of fitness through exercise and nutritional eating.

To do this I would suggest that you follow the advice I have given you in my book so far. But wait, I'm not through yet. You will continue to watch your weight to see that it remains fairly constant. You don't have to be a fanatic about this and weigh yourself every day; twice a week is more than enough. It will be up to you to balance the amount of exercise you get with the amount of your food intake. Remember, you have to achieve a sensible balance.

If you are a middle-aged woman who has a family, I would urge you to start your children on the program from their very tender years. Most children have very supple and agile bodies, but some tend to be overweight from the time they are first in your arms. You will not be doing your children any favors by stuffing them full of formula. Follow your pediatrician's suggestions carefully and don't overfeed your children. As far as exercise is concerned, I don't expect a two-month-old baby to start pelvic rolls, shoulder thrusts, and the like, but you can exercise its legs and other parts of its body by slowly and carefully moving them for a few minutes a day. As they grow older, they will be able to follow you as you do your exercises. As they mature, they can take the initiative. Any child who has followed my exercises and eating pattern from infancy has to be ahead of the game in the final analysis. It is much easier to train the body from a tender age to avoid candies filled with refined sugars and other unhealthy foods.

I have seen the difference that proper nutrition and adequate exercises have made on the children of friends of mine. The families that have been careful and have given their children healthy, nutritional foods have brought up fine, robust, and healthy children. It's incredible how much energy their children have.

I particularly admire Carrie M. and her family. They are always on the go, participating in mostly outdoor activities. They can survive winters that many of us would not get through without contracting some form of cold bug. They didn't develop this healthiness accidentally. They take very good care of their bodies, eat the right foods, get enough sleep, and exercise their minds and bodies constantly. And I have never seen any of the children eating candy.

A few years ago I introduced Carrie's family to Middle Eastern foods. They were more inclined towards natural foods at the time, so I showed them that the Middle Eastern kitchen has a great deal of "natural" foods that are filled with nutrients. They caught on very quickly, and Mrs. M. is now quite an authority on the subject.

Needless to say, they do not have a weight problem. The children are very interested in my dancing career, and I see one potential professional dancer in the bunch. Carrie M. often stays behind with me to take an Oriental dance lesson when the family is off conquering some uncharted trail. She is even teaching baby Liz some steps.

So now we come back to you. Are you going to become an Oriental dancer? No? Well, that's okay. Remember, that was not your primary goal. You reached your primary goal of shedding a certain amount of excess pounds and starring at your very own Arabian Nights party.

How do you go on from there? It is very easy. Don't let that party go to your head unless you want to become an active participant in the Oriental dance world. Then I would advise you to enroll in a dance studio that prides itself on turning out a truly professional product. Hard work and intensive training are the only means to achieve professional status. Remember, though, that you can achieve the *health* and *beauty* of an Oriental dancer without becoming a professional dancer.

Since your body is a system of thousands of interconnected parts—very vital organs and networks of veins, arteries, muscles and bones—and just like an intricate watch mechanism or any complex machine such as an automobile, you too have to have your regular tune-ups and cleaning. Your tune-up consists of a visit to your doctor from time to time to see how your body is doing. Your body needs may change, and you want to be prepared. If you have become adept at measuring your own body needs, then keep a fervent lookout for any danger signals—either of undernourishing or of overnourishing yourself. You don't have to wait until you experience a serious illness before you go to your doctor for a checkup. See your doctor regularly, even if you are feeling well. Maybe he can detect something that you cannot as a novice detect. Your doctor is thoroughly familiar with your body, and he can advise you accordingly. Remember, you want to continue on the road to good health and not fall by the wayside.

Now that you have achieved the goal that most Oriental dancers have achieved through their art, you must continue on this path. I would like to give you a list of important overall things that should become part of your lifelong pattern:

1. Maintain good posture.
2. Exercise daily.
3. Eat nutritiously prepared foods.
4. Take a daily bath or shower.
5. Have a facial massage at least once a week.

6. Have a body massage at least once a week.
7. Indulge in a manicure and pedicure at least once a week.
8. Get plenty of rest.
9. Dress attractively.
10. Apply makeup sparingly but attractively.
11. Think love and sex.

Remember what I said about posture in the beginning of the book. I expect you to maintain good posture at all times; no slouching that will leave your joints and muscles wishing they were on someone who would treat them more kindly. Your stretching exercises will help you achieve a better posture. Keep your head up, shoulders back, chest wide, stomach in, and hips relaxed at all times.

The Oriental dance exercises are a physical fitness program for you to execute daily in the privacy of your home. When you feel more confident with yourself you could enroll in an Oriental dance school. Go to several until you find one that stresses the exercise value of the dance as opposed to a school that trains professional dancers, even though the latter will have the same benefits. The difference is that when you are being trained to become a professional there are more rigorous routines that have to be followed plus intricate choreography. When you do it for the exercise value, you concentrate more on your bodily benefits. You have to separate the two goals, even though the method may be virtually the same.

Now that you have a new figure, you should want the world to see it. Your beauty is coming from within. However, I would suggest that you go beyond this and treat yourself to a makeup analysis. Salons are advertised all over the place. There you can get your facials and learn how to apply your makeup more artfully and exotically. The Cleopatra look is exciting. This outward approach to beauty should never be the be-all and end-all of everything. Remember, beauty starts from the inside. This outside touch-up adds a little spark to your life, but don't count on it to cover up internal problems.

A good facial should be the start of any makeup program. Follow the directions that I have given you in Chapter 9. When selecting your makeup, keep your skin type (dry or oily) in mind. You should also use your makeup to enhance your features. Indeed, you should use your makeup so that your face doesn't seem made up. The only time I use heavy makeup, false eyelashes and all is when I have to appear on stage, because stage makeup is needed so that Mrs. X in the last row of a large room can see you better if your features are accentuated. The bright stage lights drain all color from your face, so you must therefore make your features appear to be bigger than life.

A good cosmetic used throughout the Middle East is kohl, which is a natural product that dates back to ancient times and is even mentioned in the Qur'an. In many parts of the Middle East, such as Morocco, even men use kohl on their eyes. They use it to help cleanse their eyes of impurities rather than for the cosmetic effect.

Facials

In Chapter 9 I have given you a little insight into the types of facials that I use. Because most Oriental dancers wear a great deal of stage makeup, it is important that they take care of their skin. The best way to take care of your face is to see that it is thoroughly cleansed at all times. Whenever you wash your face, wash it with a mild soap, using warm water to open the pores so that the dirt and grime can be washed away, then rinse it with cool water to close the pores. This stimulation and cleansing of the pores will promote a clean skin. When you are home be sure to cleanse your face thoroughly of all makeup, no matter how late you come home or how tired you are.

At one of the Oriental dance workshops in New York City I was fortunate to meet the beautiful and gracious Middle Eastern dancer Elona. I was so fascinated by her demonstration of makeup for the dance that I asked her to write it for my book. Here is some advice from Elona:

> To create exotic eye makeup for the stage, first cover eye area completely with foundation, then apply powder. Then using a sable brush, a tiny sponge applicator, a cotton swab, or even fingers if they are nimble, apply color to the entire eye area including eye area underneath lower lashes (about ¼ inch) and extend beyond eye toward temple, tapering to a soft point. Choose a color to match your own eyes or complement your costume. It will look like a triangle of color from the inner corner of the eye and tapering out toward the hairline.
>
> Next, use a high shimmer powder in white, silver, gold, or pale pink to heighten underneath the brow. Carry this highlight color out to the temples, following the line of the triangle, meeting at the point near the temple. Using the same light highlighter, touch the top of the eyelid, just above the iris and close to the lashline, creating a dot of highlight there.
>
> For contrast and depth, choose a very dark matte color

(such as powdered eyebrow makeup) in either dark brown or deep charcoal and now create a natural shadow by shading this dark color just above the eyelid in the crease of the eye. Shape it in an arc of deep shadow, like a crescent, and blend it out to the point near the temple. Blend these three colors together at the edges by gently rubbing back and forth with the applicator. Use a different applicator for each of these colors for more control. The effect is one of natural highlights and shadows just as an artist would use to draw an eye with depth on paper.

Eyeliner in black or deep brown is next applied from the inner corner of the eye at the base of the upper lashline and extending beyond the eye to the same point at the temple. Consider the winged effect desired by always tapering the eyeliner to end in delicate points . . . upward and outward. Fill in the lower lash toward the cheeks. Use one strong line and alternate with two lighter ones, continuing these strokes toward the inner corner of the eye, stopping with a dot.

False eyelashes can then be applied to the upper and lower lashes. Use a thick fringe of lash for the upper and delicate spikes for the lower. The total effect is darkly dramatic and this entire procedure can be adapted for daytime wear by using a lighter hand. Do everything the same way but with a lighter touch and modify the triangle color extension.

For a festive touch, place a small dot of spirit gum to the inner corners of the eye and touch tiny sparkle star gently in place with tweezers. Light colors, pinks and red look best.

For extremely exotic Egyptian eyes, an artistic hand or lots of practice is needed! This takes time and a steady hand. Prop the elbow on a table top. Apply eye makeup the same way only change the eyeliner and draw a thick heavy line (about ¼ inch) from the inner corner of upper eyelid out toward temples, following the triangle of color. This technique does not end in a delicate point, but rather a squared end. It is also extended out toward the temples a bit further than normal liner. Heavy liner is applied also under the lower lashes and extended out to meet the top line. The eyebrows are elongated and extend out to the temples ending in a blunt squared off line also. The end of the brow is directly over the end of the eyeliner and they appear parallel. Egyptian eyes are suitable for distance viewing and tribal-type costumes. For a finishing touch, a pseudo-tattoo can be drawn on the face on the cheekbone. Use black waterproof liner and draw four square dots in a tiny horizontal diamond shape directly under one eye on the cheekbone. The ancient people felt this warded away evil spirits. Henna on the palms of the hands was also used for this purpose.

Hair

Thorough brushing of your hair stimulates the scalp and thus the secretion of natural oils, which is very good for maintaining healthy hair. Your hair should always be combed properly—from the end of the hair first, down the strand of hair until you get to your scalp. A healthy scalp will start a healthy head of hair.

Your hair should be styled to suit your face. Most dancers have long hair because it is more exciting to see a head of hair flowing with the movements of the dancer's body, but you need not become hung up over long hair. There are many attractive wigs available for the purpose. You should be careful with these and wear them judiciously so that you give your hair time to breathe. I killed my hair wearing wigs when I first started dancing. From time to time you can wrap a scarf around your head in an imaginative way. You often see the older women in the Middle East, Greece, and Turkey with their heads wrapped in scarves. There are some charming scarves available from that part of the world that have small coins on the edges. A rinse of henna, which is a natural Middle Eastern product, will give your hair a lovely touch of color. I also understand that it is very good for the hair and much better than those artificial dyes.

Scalp Massage

This section of the body needs just as much "exercise" as any other part of your body. You can exercise your scalp by massaging it. The simplest form of massage is brushing the hair. This process stretches the skin and stimulates the blood vessels and nerves, thus promoting a healthy, lively scalp. The massage should be done by a professional; however, I'll list here a few simple ones that I learned in yoga and elsewhere. You should be able to do these easily:

1. Grab hold of the roots of the hair near the scalp in the front of your head. Pull the hair gently but firmly forward and backward, repeating this motion five or six times. You should feel your scalp moving while doing this.
2. Start at the middle of the back of the skull. Take your fingers and, in a rotating motion, move up the neck. Continue around the side of your head until you reach the center forehead. Repeat twice.
3. Take both hands and hold your head gently but firmly. The thumbs should be in the middle of the base of the skull.

Fingers are up over your ears. Slide the fingers back and forth gently so as to move the scalp.

Some of the ancient hair styles fascinate me. The ancient Egyptian hair style was a very short bob, usually with bangs, and sometimes the hair was straight and sometimes it was even very frizzy. The ancient Greek hair style was wavy and pulled back in a sort of bun. Today it seems that, with the jet age upon us, there doesn't seem to be much difference between the hair styles throughout the world. The only difference I have found is that more Middle Eastern women wear their hair long and don't fuss about beauty parlors as much as American or, on a lesser scale, European women.

Body Massage

I would recommend that you get a professional massage at least once a week. Of course if you want to economize a little, train someone in your family to give you a massage. There are books available on the subject.

You may ask yourself, "Why massage?" Well, have you had one lately? It is the greatest and should be used in your lifelong program of physical fitness. It should never be used in place of physical exercise, because excessive fat will not disappear by thumping it away. Massage can help such things as a double chin or fat on the back of your arms disappear. Massage helps your muscles feel better; it doesn't build strength like the Oriental dance exercises do. A massage will help to smoothe out the wrinkles and extra folds that may appear when you lose a great deal of weight.

The purpose of a massage is to speed up circulation, which will in turn speed up all your normal bodily processes. Respiration and excretion are greatly helped. A massage will stimulate reflex action in the nerves. It causes a healthy glow of your skin and stimulates activity of the glands and other organs. It forces blood through the body of the muscles, thus causing an increased blood supply to them, which improves the nutrition of the muscles and makes them firm and elastic. It revitalizes the muscles without exhausting them, and it removes fatigue from the muscles and leaves them in good condition. Your digestion will also be improved through the stimulation of nerves in the digestive organs.

Through massage you will get a sense of well-being. The stroking motions relieve nervous irritation and ease pain, and therefore help you to relax. The oils used can help your body to feel soft and smooth all over.

When you are being massaged you should be completely relaxed. It helps if the person who's giving you the massage is at peace with himself and is full of energy, because that person can then transfer this energy through his fingertips to your body. Have I given you enough reasons why you should have an occasional massage? I certainly hope so.

When you get your massage, let the person who is doing it start at the top of your head and work all the way to the tips of your toes. Don't let a spot be missed. One of my feet is all messed up because of an operation I had, and after a show there is nothing that helps ease the pain better than a good foot massage.

Clothes

The Middle Eastern look in clothing is definitely with us. Previously, only the expensive boutiques carried these exotic items—at, I might add, exotic prices. Nowadays I have seen them in the department stores around town at very reasonable prices. Of course they can be found in most Oriental dance boutiques. Some of the designs are quite sexy looking, and believe me you do not have to be naked to be sexy, but they have a certain alluring look to them. You should buy some loose-fitting kaftans or galabayas to wear for lounging around the house, but I would advise you to get some more form-fitting designs that will show off your figure for those special nights. If you are married you will become more attractive to your husband; if not, you will look good for that special beau of yours; and if neither of the aforementioned is the case, you will certainly be alluring to yourself and any number of unsuspecting people.

Love and Sex

Somehow I have managed to leave love and sex out of this book up to now, but what book would be successful without some sex thrown in? Seriously, though, you have heard the question, "Do Oriental dancers have more fun sexually?" It used to be the blondes, now it is the Oriental dancers. This is a very hard question to answer in a few paragraphs, but I would like to sum it up by saying, yes, they do. I think that because they have spent years perfecting their art, respecting their bodies and their capabilities, and they have come to the point where they can shower that sexual feeling on someone else, that they tend to have healthy sex lives. I haven't yet met a dancer who wasn't a warm sensitive human being.

You, through the Oriental dance exercises and a nutritionally sound eating program, have freed your body of all the knots that were binding it and inhibiting it from performing as it should sexually. A supple body is the key to healthy sexual activity. It also takes a willing and cooperative partner, and to find one you will have to exude a certain special something that will provoke a mate's sensitivity and sensualness.

Beware, though, because there is no such thing as taking ten Oriental dance lessons and launching a career as a fantastic lover the next day! The idea that I am trying to bring across goes much deeper than that. You have to work at being a good lover, and just as you work at nurturing your inner self, you must work at nurturing your sexual self with an attitude that will bring you to new heights sexually. There is no doubt that Oriental dancing has a sexual aura built around it. It is therefore up to you to build a positive sexual aura rather than a negative sexual aura around yourself through the dance.

Some people choose to ignore this aspect of the dance, but I choose to bring it out into the open and discuss it in a positive manner. In case you hadn't noticed, sex is here to stay, and the sooner you start discussing it sensibly and taking the ugliness out of it, the sooner you will lead sexually fulfilling lives. It would serve you well to heed the poet, Khalil Gibran's words about sex:

> The most highly sexed beings upon the planet are the creators, the poets, sculptors, painters, musicians . . . and so it has been from the beginning. And among them sex is a beautiful and exalted gift. Sex is always beautiful. And, it is always shy.*

This book has shown you some of the ways that you can develop this whole new attitude toward yourself and ultimately toward sex. Keep that positive attitude about yourself going at all times. Just as you were able to take off your excess weight, so you are also capable of doing many other things with your body if you put your mind to it. You will achieve anything you want to achieve by freeing your mind, your body, and your soul. You, and only you, can make things happen if you have a positive attitude toward yourself. Get all those "I can't" thoughts out of your head. You can do it. Think positively. Think sex. Allow the Oriental dancing to help you on your way.

Just the other day I was talking to a friend of mine who teaches dance, and she mentioned many of her students whom she had helped find new lives through the dance. She told me about a woman

*The Wisdom of Gibran, edited by Joseph Sheban, Philosophical Library, Inc., 15 East 40th Street, N.Y. 10016. Copyright © 1966.

who came to take lessons from her after her husband had died. It took her a lot of courage to get this far; however, she still was not able to get back into the swing of things—she felt alone and started to withdraw from life. My friend was very positive with her, and little by little this woman got involved with the dance until one night my friend invited her to accompany her to one of her performances. At this outing the woman met a very nice gentleman, and four months later they are still seeing each other.

Up to this point in my book I have been showing you how to become a more sensitive human being. I haven't said it in so many words, but the implications are there because, if your body is in tiptop shape, you begin feeling better about yourself, and this glow is bound to show before long. These wishes will be transmitted to others around you, and since ladies usually like the attention of the opposite sex, new relationships are bound to blossom. I have done an informal survey regarding which one of the real "me" would get more attention from the other sex. Most times I do not tell people right out that I am an Oriental dancer. I tell them that I am a public school teacher, and as the conversation progresses, I merely drop the information that I am also an Oriental dancer. With few exceptions, this always makes men, and even women, more interested in me.

Let me now give you some more specific ideas that you may want to use to "turn on" that special person. Let us start with the perfumes. The exotic perfumes of the Middle East have always fascinated me. Perfumes were very important to the people of Egypt. Myrrh, which is an aromatic, resinous exudation from certain plants of the genus *commiphora*, especially myrrha, a shiny shrub, was used extensively in the Middle East for incense, perfumes, and in medicine. The three magi brought the child Jesus gifts of gold, frankincense, and myrrh. It was also used in Egypt for embalming corpses—not too pleasant a thought but nevertheless interesting. When archaeologist Howard Carter discovered the tomb of the boy king Tutankhamen, he found at least 50 jars of different kinds of unguents there.

You should be aware that, even today, for example, Moroccan women, when they attend the Hamadsha curing ceremony, will practically bathe themselves in perfumes. This is the occasion when they perform their trance dance or guedra (hadra). This is one of the few times when women are permitted to dance while men are present. Most women dance only for each other. If you dance in the presence of men, somehow you are supposed to lose your respectability.

You must learn how to use these scents and aromas to your advantage. The only time that I "bathe" in perfume, but never to an overpowering degree, is when I am performing. I always use a good perfume, because one doesn't want to permeate a "cheap" scent through the audience. I find that "sexy" aromas permeating through an audience add to the mystique of the dance. One of the owners of a hotel where I work quite a bit always kids me about my perfumes. He swears that he can smell me a mile away. He says that he never has to see me before a show to know that I am there, because he can always smell my scent around the place. Most places like to know that a performer has shown up on time for rehearsals and a performance so that they don't have to get ulcers trying to book another act at the last minute in case you don't show. So you see, my perfume helps to prevent some ulcers!

Off stage it is not "chic" to use too much of a strong perfume. I find that subtle smells are very, very sexy, and you should make sure that your perfume is not offensive. Too strong an odor can sometimes irritate your sinuses, and ultimately someone who doesn't like that smell as much as you do. There are some lovely oils that cling nicely to your skin which you can purchase in some of the ethnic stores around town. Check them out.

The Berbers of Morocco have a great way to achieve a pleasant smell. Actually the process they use is not done for cosmetic purposes but rather as a sort of superstition. They wear belts around their waists which have puffs of fabric filled with spices. These are none other than sachets of glorious scents in them, such as cloves, jasmin, roses, iris, and mint. The scent of these crushed herbs is supposed to ward off evil spirits. These bands are also used around the head and busts. The Dades roses from the valley of Mgouna, Morocco are simply ethereal. Some of the other great smells of Morocco include the narcissuses, gerberas, iris, and mimosas. Some other popular aromas of the Middle East are amber, sandalwood, lily of the valley, orange blossom, and lavender.

A Moroccan friend of mine has been making some of these scented belts, American style, and I find them to be quite sexy. You achieve a constant beautiful aroma to your being. It surely beats having to replenish your faded perfume aroma from time to time. Take a little hint from the Berbers and wrap yourself in some exotic scent.

It is hard for me to talk about things that supposedly will make you sexy, because I think of sex as a very personal thing, and besides that, I am not writing a sexual manual as I don't feel that I am such an expert on the subject. I have given it a lot of thought, however, and I just had to share my thoughts with you.

It is the nature of the Oriental dance business to have men think of us as sexual objects. Most dancers find this annoying because they want their art, rather than their sexiness, to be appreciated in a positive manner. Furthermore, I think that men pay attention to any attractive girl who happens to come their way, whether she is wearing an Oriental dance costume or basic secretarial garb. Of course when one is on stage in a brief cabaret costume, the aura of sex burns even brighter, and more than the normal man-woman attraction develops. This is a natural occurrence but I think it should be kept in its perspective. In fact there is many a time when I try very hard to show a low profile when I am on a job and some guy is playing up to Lebwa the Oriental dancer rather than Lebwa the woman.

Without stepping foot on a stage, you too can help brighten that sexual aura around you by developing an exotic look. Most men are attracted to women who have a mystical look about them, and what better to have than that *exotic* look of the Oriental dancer and the Middle East. Remember it wasn't too long ago that the women there went around with only their eyes showing. Even today that custom is still practiced in Saudi Arabia and other more religious outposts of the Arab world. Many other Middle Eastern countries may have shed this custom, but their women still believe in perpetuating that mystique. You don't find them flaunting their bodies in public.

One of the most common forms of dress for Middle Eastern women is called a kaftan. These are long dresses, sometimes intricately embroidered, that cover everything. They are just as sexy, if not sexier, than any plunging necklines you could wear. Many of the women do dress in the Western mode these days; however, that Middle Eastern touch is still there. This look has finally caught on here, and you can get kaftans and the like in just about any store.

Many Oriental dance boutiques have sprung up all over the United States, and besides stocking the usual Oriental dance costumes these shops have rather nice Middle Eastern jewelry, kaftans, belledi dresses and the like. Start with a small piece of jewelry, and as time goes by you can add to your wardrobe. In time you'll be looking very exotic, and you will be attracting a lot of new friends. You'll have a lot to say about your new-found look.

After you have mastered some of the Oriental dance exercises and you have "come out" at that Arabian Nights party for your friends, give your husband or that special someone a private showing. Then you don't have to wonder about what that certain Oriental dancer had that made everyone's eyes pop open. You'll find out very fast.

You don't have to get involved with any new sexual techniques. Sexual techniques depend upon the happiness you derive from a happy sexual relationship. You don't need to be taught sex. It just happens. You won't find it in a book. If your body is in shape you will be able to enjoy yourself more.

The sexual drive should be distinguished from what we call love. When you love someone, you perceive something to be unique in that person. Sex and love are by no means the same thing. The two do go very well together. However, love is an emotion, sex is not an emotion—it is conceived as a sensation. It's up to you to differentiate between the two. It's up to you to know when to settle down from all the new sensations of sex to the seriousness of love. In ancient times in the Middle East people didn't engage in either love or sex as we know them today. No one got married because they were in love. Your partner was chosen for you, and that was that. Since sex comes naturally, it wasn't hard to have offspring, and they did this all without the latest sex manual of the day. This sort of "arrangement" still goes on today, however, in a much more informal way.

Music

Now that we have gotten sex out of the way, let's talk about the musical world of the Oriental dancer. This is a very special one and one with which you should become thoroughly familiar because it can help to heighten your sensitivity. Middle Eastern music is played with a great deal of subjectivity in that the performers are always adding their own embellishments to the written music. The music is played with passion and a great deal of sensuality, producing a sound that literally overwhelms the senses. The poet, Khalil Gibran sums up my feelings about music so splendidly:

> The moaning flute is more divine than the golden cup of deep, red wine . . . God created music as a common language for all men. It inspires the poets, the composers and the architects. It lures us to search our souls for the meaning of the mysteries described in ancient books . . . When God created Man he gave him Music as a language different from all other languages. And early man sang her glory in the wilderness, and she drew the hearts of kings and moved them from their thrones.*

When I listen to the hypnotic music of the Middle East, I get a satisfying feeling that transports me close to the point of intoxication, and speaking of sex, the music is almost as good! The Greek word for this feeling is "kefi." The Arabs call if "kef." In the United States I

*The Wisdom of Gibran, edited by Joseph Sheban, Philosophical Library, Inc., 15 East 40th Street, N.Y. 10016. Copyright © 1966.

suppose we would say, "heavy, man, heavy." When the music reaches an appreciative audience, you can hear them crying out such words as "Allah" or "Maşallah," which is the Turkish way of saying "wonderful," "God bless you," or "What wonders God hath willed." You too can make this music a part of your life.

Middle Eastern music is sometimes hard to appreciate when you first hear it, because it is played in quarter tones which are hard for the American or European ear to understand. It will be necessary to educate your ear to really get to appreciate music that is so different from Western music. Arabic music is a constant repetition of one or two fundamental sounds on which a melodic idea is heard. One classical example of repetition in Arabic music and song was when the great Egyptian singer Um Kalthoum performed at a concert and sang one verse over fifty times, each of these times gaining increased momentum and tonation, and carried her audience into ecstasy. Her phrasing would turn a simple phrase, sung over and over, into a glorious musical experience.

Even the spoken word in the Middle East has a beautiful tonal quality. In the mosques of the Middle East and Turkey one can hear the almost musical recitation of the Qur'an taking place. I am always amazed at how beautifully musical these recitations are. I had an Arab friend who was devoutly religious, and I would sit spellbound when he would pray. Um Kalthoum used to sing the Qur'an verses when she was young. There is a story that, because of the Islamic view of women, when she was a young girl, she would have to dress up in boy's clothing in order to sing in the mosque. The call to prayer, which is the Islamic way of summoning the faithful, is a beautiful chant. The Muezzin calls out, "Allahu Akbar" (God is most great) from the minaret of the mosque. The faithful are called to prayer five times a day—dawn, midday, mid-afternoon, sunset, and nightfall.

Classical music was the music "accepted" by the world of Islam, although the Qur'an forbids music. The prophet Mohammed in his teachings had condemned the study and use of music because of all the seeming decadence that was carried on in the places where music was played.

The Arabs, through their armies, picked up some of the musical instruments from other countries as they crisscrossed them. The oud, for instance, came from Persia. We don't get to hear too much of the classical music, and just as well, because it is more difficult than the music associated with the Oriental dance for the Western ear to absorb. The music we hear today is the folk music of the sailors, fishermen, camel drivers, the wedding songs, and the plaintive strains of the funeral dirges rather than the classical music. At most of the Arabic festivities, entertainment is provided by songs in which the emphasis is placed on the words and beautiful repetitious melody rather than on the music.

Arabic music has a kind of persistent quality played in a quarter-tone scale, and emphasis is placed on the melody rather than on the rhythm. Arabic music, like many other customs of that part of the world, has been unchanged for centuries. Middle Eastern music has many diverse musical traditions, such as Turkish, Arabic, and Persian. The Arabic tradition can be divided into three areas: Syrian, Iraqi, and Egyptian. They are all related in some way. Early Arabic musicians possibly were wandering minstrels like those we read of in the Arabian Nights. They were as much poets as they were musicians. In fact, the Arab songs are usually poems that have been set to music. In the world of Islam it is vocal music that reigns supreme.

A brief mention should be made here of Armenian music. This area is often referred to as the Russian Middle East. From the seventh to the ninth centuries Armenia was under Arab domination. Turkey and Persia also occupied this territory. Alexander the Great conquered it during the fourth century. If you recall, the Arabs were in central Asia from the end of the eighth century. Many of the instruments used in Armenian music are typically Middle Eastern. The nai and the rebab are two of them.

You should become familiar with the instruments pictured in this chapter. Many of these instruments are used in various combinations to form an orchestra that can back an Oriental dancer. A Greek orchestra may be very different from a Turkish or Arabic orchestra. Today in many of the ethnic clubs you can hear all types of music being played, such as Greek, Israeli, Turkish, and Arabic. The audiences demand this and will shout out for their favorite requests. If the audience is mixed, the music will be mixed so that everyone is satisfied. If there is a preponderance of one ethnic group then you will hear that music. The club owners are very cognizant of the fact that they have to cater to the dominant group of customers.

Unfortunately, a dancer does not always have the use of an authentic orchestra and sometimes has to work with an American orchestra that plays a few traditional folk dances such as "Miserlou" and "Hava Nageela." This is a very limiting experience for a dancer. If there is anything that can turn a dancer off, it's having to dance to an orchestra that does not play authentic Middle Eastern music. In the Middle East the necessary importance is placed on the orchestra that plays for a dancer. There are even original pieces written exclusively for dancers. I believe that Nadia Gamal was one of the first dancers to be honored in this special way.

Soon dancers will be able to go anywhere and have their music played for them, thanks to some enterprising musicians who have finally seen fit to write out some of the more typical Oriental dance music so that any orchestra can play it. We dancers still have a long way to go because most hotels will not hire extra authentic musicians for a dancer. They figure that they have an orchestra, let the girl use that. One of the alternatives for Oriental dancers is to insist that orchestras read and play their music, and now they have the tool to use—written Oriental dance music. A friend of mine had several charts made for me a long time ago, but the ironic thing is that many of the bands I worked with could not play the music anyway.

Some funny moments have been associated with the musicians I have had to work with over the years. Once I had to dance to the music of a solo organist who had never played for a performer. The only place he had ever played was in church on Sunday. Can you imagine the "prayers" I had to say during that performance! Two other funny times were when I had to work with a Spanish orchestra just off the plane from San Juan, Puerto Rico, and when I was confronted with an orchestra that played only big band jazz music. To the latter musicians, even such standard tunes as "Caravan," "Hava Nageela", and "Fiddler on the Roof" seemed like ancient times. All the musicians could say was, "Like man, we don't play that. Can you dance to 'Take the A Train'?"

Egyptian music dates back to about the fourth millenium B.C. In the Egyptian tombs you can see paintings of male and female musicians playing their instruments. For example, female musicians are clearly depicted in the tomb of Nakht (1415 B.C.) at Thebes, Egypt.

Turkish music is a sort of Persian-Arabic music. It is mostly folk, military, and religious music, as you would find in most Islamic cultures.

Geographically, Greece is part of Europe, but it's hard for me to separate it from the ancient Middle East. Ancient Greek music was linked to the poetry of the time. Historians have found ancient Greek music written in the Greek alphabet rather than the musical notation to which we are accustomed. In fact, the Greeks have left us a great deal of evidence of their music. On Greek vases you can see pictures of instruments clearly. You can see scenes from religious rites, the theater, and mythology. In keeping with the Greek mind, music was considered an art as well as a science. The Greeks even developed a system of scales and intervals.

You should visit some of the Greek, Israeli, and Middle Eastern nightclubs in your area and feast your mind, body, and soul on the ecstatic sounds of those areas. This is the only "feast" in which you'll be allowed to partake—you won't gain any weight this way—so go ahead and fill your ears with the music of the Oriental dancer. Numerous instruments are used in the folk music of the Middle East, Greece, and Turkey. I have illustrated and described the most important ones here for you.

Bouzoukee (Buzuki)

This is the chordophone of modern Greece. It was introduced to Greece and Turkey about the beginning of the twentieth century. It is a pot-bellied lute with a long fretted neck. It has steel strings which are played with a pick. It is the most popular instrument of Greece.

At one time, "nice" people in Greece did not frequent the bouzoukee bistros because the music was considered indigenous to lower-class people (as our jazz used to be regarded). It was popular in the waterfront cafes of Salonika and Piraeus. Most of the songs dealt with lost loves, loneliness, unfaithfulness, sailors longing for their homeland, and the joys of smoking hashish.

Bouzoukee music was suppressed in Greece until after World War II, and then it was brought out into the open. It became popular in America after an article was written in the newspapers about New

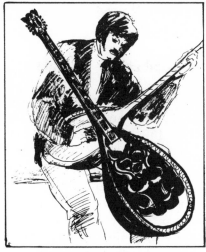

Bouzoukee (Buzuki)

York's Eighth Avenue Greek clubs that featured Oriental dancers. The impetus from the movies "Never on Sunday" and "Zorba the Greek" gave the bouzoukee its push to stardom, and today the bouzoukee is synonymous with Greece.

Def (Duff)

This is an Egyptian tambourine inlaid with mother of pearl. The Albanians use a form of this instrument, which is a frame drum with cymbals attached to it. This is played mostly by women.

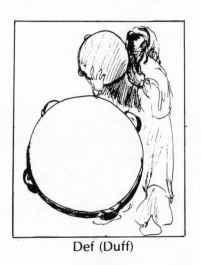

Def (Duff)

Derbeke (Dumbeg, Dumbeck or Durbakki)

The derbeke is an Arabic drum that has a cone or cylindrical shape like a goblet and a thin layer of dried sheepskin or fish skin stretched across the top. In North America the cone is made of clay. The most modern ones, especially in the Middle East, are made of copper, although they are also made of pottery. It is more popular with the musicians who play folk music; however, this instrument is also used for classical music. The Persian model of this drum has more inlaid work typical of that country. Depending on the size, it can be held under the arm or between the legs. It is played with both hands: the fingers of the right hand strike the head of the drum, more forcibly than the fingers of the left hand, which usually play around the rim of the drum, sometimes in a snapping form of motion.

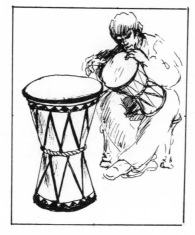

Derbeke (Dumbeg, Dumbec, or Durbakki)

Kanun (Kanoun)

The kanun is a plucked chordophone and may be referred to as the Middle Eastern harp or zither, except that it is much smaller than the harp. The basic difference is that it is held horizontally in the player's lap as he or she plucks its double strings with both hands. Four to eight nail tips made of whalebone or quills, fastened by rings, are used on the player's index fingers. This instrument has 26 metal strings, and it makes some of the sweetest sounds this side of heaven. It is of Turkish origin, but it is also widely used in the Middle East and Greece.

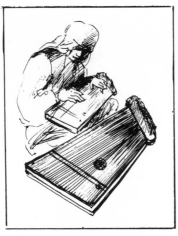

Kanun (Kanoun)

Kemache (Kamanja or Kemenche)

This is a violin-type instrument of Persian origin. It is a bowed chordophone that has a small round body, often made of coconut, with a long neck. The coconut is pierced with a spike, on which the instrument rests next to the seated player. The musician holds the instrument on his or her knee. It has two to four strings of hair which are played with a primitive type of bow. In Egypt, the belly of the instrument is made of fish skin. Today it is played throughout the Arab-speaking world and in Turkey, but it is extinct in the Maghreb.

This instrument is similar to the rebab, another bowed chordophone which is used in Egypt and Turkey, except that the rebab has only one string and may be shaped a little differently.

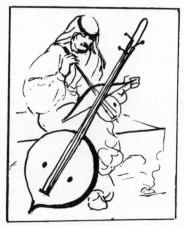

Kemache (Kamanja or Kemenche)

Nai (Nay)

The nai is probably the oldest Arab instrument in use today. It is also a Turkish instrument. In the course of its history, the nai has come to be many things in many places. It is a simple reed flute that originated in Egypt many thousands of years ago. It is now in use from Egypt to Persia. It is a vertical bamboo flute, about two feet long, with nine joints and no blowing tip. There are seven holes altogether. Two holes are placed in the second joint, two in the third, two in the fourth, and one on the opposite side of the fifth joint of the bamboo. We also find this kind of flute in the Balkan states and in Turkey, especially in Anatolia, as well as in the Arab countries. The gypsies of Yugoslavia, especially Macedonia, play this flute. They call it the kaval and the Greeks call it the kavala. The kaval is made of wood and has one additional hole on each side of it. There is also an Egyptian bamboo flute that is similar to the nai called the argal.

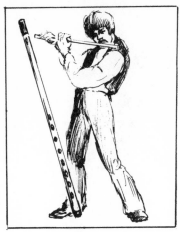

Nai (Nay)

Oud (Outi, Ud)

The oud, or Arabic lute, is a plucked chordophone known as the father of the guitar. It originated in Persia, although some people think that it came from Spain. It is a pot-bellied instrument resembling an overgrown watermelon with a short curved neck. It is made of wood and has five pairs of strings which are plucked with a plectrum, quill, or pick. The Laghouto oud (Greek bouzoukee) has a straight long neck and four double strings with metal frets. The oud has a beautiful, deep mellow tone. It is often used as a solo instrument to create improvisational wonders. It is known as the lauta in Turkey and the gosha in Mauretania. In the Balkans it is still called the ud or uti. The oud does not have frets. It is therefore easier to improvise without the medium of notes. Its descendents are the lute and mandolin. This is one of the most beautiful of Arabic instruments. It can be made very simply without elaborate designs; however, some ouds have the most beautifully intricate designs I have ever seen on an instrument. In Egypt they call this instrument the kvitarah.

Saz

This is a Persian and Turkish instrument. It is in the family of plucked chordophones of modern Anatolia and resembles a long-necked lute. It has a small body, long neck, sixteen movable frets, and a variable number of strings. The family comprises the following members: cura saz, baglama, lozuk, achik saz, and meydan saz. There is a slightly different version used in Armenia and Azerbaijan.

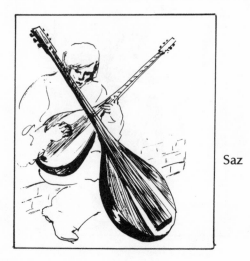

Saz

Tabla (Tabl)

The tabla is also called the tempo or tamparin. It is said that it originated in Damascus, Syria. It is a cylindrical drum that can be made of wood, metal, or clay in the shape of two truncated cones joined at their narrowest parts.

Tambourine

The tambourine is the same percussion instrument that you see in any American orchestra. It is a shallow frame drum of Middle

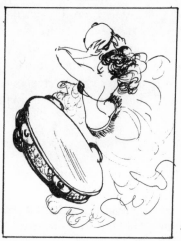

Tambourine

Eastern origin that was reintroduced to Europe with eighteenth century Turkish music. Metal jingles, two inches in diameter, are inserted in holes cut into the frame. It may be played with the fingers or with closed knuckles, or simply shaken so that one hears the jingles ringing. The tambourine used in the Middle East is usually larger and has more cymbals on it. It is used extensively by the gypsies in the Middle East and played mostly by women.

Violin

The violin is the same popular version as the violin we see in American or European orchestras, except that it is tuned differently—in fourths instead of fifths—to facilitate the numerous Arabic scales that require quarter-tones.

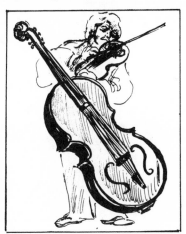

Violin

Wooden Spoons

A set of four spoons used by Turkish women in a manner similar to Spanish castanets were a predecessor to the zills (see next section). In many Egyptian tomb paintings, the dancers are seen hitting pieces of wood together. One can see wooden spoons being used today in the folk dances of Konya, Turkey. Four spoons are used, two in each hand.

Zills

Zills are a set of four metal cymbals that vary in size from approximately one-and-a-half to three inches in diameter, with elastic loops pulled through the centers. The zills are worn on the thumbs and middle fingers of both hands and are hit together to produce a variety of sounds and rhythmic patterns.

Zills were known as cymbals in ancient and modern Islam. They were used in military music for several centuries in Turkey. Their use spread from there to the Balkan peoples and the Kurds. Today the Kurds and the Turks still call their cymbals by this name. Middle Eastern dancers use them to add an extra dimension to their dance. Most times the dancer plays the zills to accentuate the rhythms, but oftentimes she will also play a counter rhythm.

Zills are called the sunuj or nuviksat in Syria and sagat in Lebanon, Egypt, and other Middle Eastern countries.

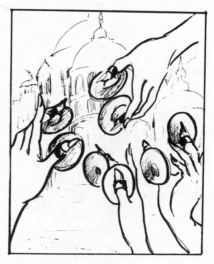

Zills

The following are some of the more popular rhythms associated with the Middle East, Turkey, and Greece.

—*Chifte Telli* is a slow 4/4 rhythm that has four beats to the measure. This is sometimes speeded up to produce a fast 4/4 rhythmic pattern.

—*Taksim* is an improvisational rhythm. It does not have a time signature. Many dancers use this for their slow, sensuous "floor work."

—*Karshlama* is a 9/8 rhythm. This is a unique Turkish rhythm that drives American orchestras crazy. A 9/8 rhythm is generally called "zeybek" in Turkey, getting its name from the zeybek folk dancers.

I love to dance and
I love to live
I hope with all of my heart
You've enjoyed what I have had to give.

May God be with you—*English*
O Theos mazi sou—*Greek*
Allah ismarladik—*Turkish*
Allah koon ma'eck—*Arabic*

appendix

MIDDLE EASTERN ORIENTAL DANCING SCHOOLS
FROM COAST TO COAST

Please note that the listings here do not in any form constitute an endorsement of a school. Schools are listed here merely for your convenience. It's an answer to your question, "Where can I take Oriental dancing lessons?" Check a school or studio thoroughly before you enroll in it.

Alabama

The Genie's Middle Eastern
Dancers
Marles, Instructor
1805 Mountain Brook Drive S.E.
Huntsville, AL 35801
(205) 533-1447

Arizona

"Electra" Karamargin's
Creative Dance Center
2802 N. Desert Avenue
Tucson, AZ 85712
(602) 881-0739 or 325-9944

Arkansas

The Mirana Studio of
Middle Eastern Dance
257 Plainview Circle
No. Little Rock, AR 72116
(501) 753-5122

California

Amina School of Belly Dancing
829 Elizabeth Street
San Francisco, CA 94114
(415) 282-7910

Jodette's Academy
P. O. Box 9024
Sacramento, CA 95816
(916) 929-8429 or 447-0637

Lakalana
3525 Beverly Glen
Sherman Oaks, CA 91403
(213) 789-0694

Sula's Belly Dance World
1235 Boulevard Way
Walnut Creek, CA 94595
(415) 937-7852

Connecticut

Bill Miller Dance Arts Center
Rte. # 1
Branford, CT 06405
(203) 488-4583

Miss Joyce School of Dance
148 Center Street
Southington, CT 06489
(203) 621-2053 or 621-5155

Miss Katherine's Dance Studio
25 Union Street
Winsted, CT 06098
(203) 379-3733

District of Columbia

Adriana's Mecca of
Middle Eastern Dance
2338 Wisconsin Avenue, N.W.
Washington, D. C. 20007
(202) 338-4525

Florida

Juliana Dance Gallery
102 Giralda
Coral Gables, FL 33134
(305) 448-6420

Veda Sereem "Art of
Belly Dancing" Studio
Seminole Plaza Shopping Center
Casselberry, FL 32707
(305) 831-1322

Georgia

Kalila
3481 Ridgecrest Drive
Powder Springs, GA 30073
(404) 943-4198

Hawaii

Shalimar
University of Hawaii
College of Continuing Education
and Student Services
2500 Dole Street
Honolulu, HI 96822
(808) 948-8866

Illinois

Barbara Cargill (Natasha)
333 Ridgewood
Glen Ellyn, IL 60137
(312) 469-4641

Dee's School of
Mid-Eastern Dance
1907 West Springfield
Champaign, IL 61820
(217) 359-3529

Lynda Gard (Bacchea)
1206 North Walnut Street
Danville, IL 61832
(217) 446-5586

Melanie Sanford
856 North Spring Street
Elgin, IL 60120
(312) 888-1103

Indiana

Darana Navel Academy of
Carmel Indiana
1503 East Riverside Drive
Indianapolis, IN 46202
(317) 846-1921

Judy Hanna Self Improvement
and Belly Dancing School
5302 North Bosart Avenue
Indianapolis, IN 46220
(317) 257-5576

Dixon Dance Studios
5845 North Haverford Street
Indianapolis, IN 46220
(317) 897-0369 (24 hours)

Zabrena School
of Mid-Eastern Dance
509 South Eddy Street
South Bend, IN 46617
(219) 232-5222

Kansas

Sahda & Mahmoud
Belly Dancing Academy
1719 Scott
Wichita, KS 67216
(316) 262-3609

Shalena's School of
Belly Dancing
1118 North Monroe
Hutchinson, KS 67501
(316) 662-3153

Maine

Clara Harnden Desjardins Studio
86 Main Street
Auburn, ME 04210
(207) 784-5942

Maryland

Patrima School of
Mid-Eastern Dance
Pat Marggraf, Director
19213 Mt. Airey Road
Brookeville, MD 20729
(301) 774-0816

Sadana Middle Eastern Ballet
19 Tynewick Ct.
Silver Spring, MD 20906
(314) 598-8771

Massachusetts

Scheherazade Studios
(Morwenna Nevitt)
13 Bisbee Street
West Wareham, MA 02576
(617) 748-1098

Shirley Baker Studios of
Oriental Belly Dance
and Rhythmic Slimnastics
60 Nardone Road
Needham, MA 02192
(617) 444-7406

Michigan

Christine Jablonski (Tina)
11724 Declerck
Sterling Heights, MI 48078
(313) 264-0159

Myrna Danse Du Ventre Atelier
15682 Lake Shore Road
P. O. Box 319, R.R.I.
Union Pier, MI 49129
(616) 469-4459 or 469-4359

Suheyla—Arts World
(Institute of Creative Arts)
213½ South Main Street
Ann Arbor, MI 48105
(313) 994-8400

Missouri

Diana's Fine Art Center
3830 Cleveland
St. Louis, MO 63110
(314) 771-5241

Opal's Belly Dance World
P. O. Box 20199
St. Louis, MO 63123
(314) 843-8282 or 843-1931

Nevada

Dalilah's International
Dance Studio
Belly Dance Studio and Boutique
3983 West Charleston Boulevard
Las Vegas, NV 89102
(702) 878-9910

New Jersey

Dance with Doris Rivera
7 Washington Place
Ramsey, NJ 07446
(201) 825-3145

Deshara's
440 Bentley Road
East Windsor, NJ 08520
(609) 443-4531

Loretta Turner Dance Studio
100 Wedgewood Drive
Cinnaminson, NJ 08077
(609) 829-3605

Mid-East School of Dance
(Penny LoBello)
81 Cortland Place
Tenafly, NJ 07670
(201) 569-2225

The Nani Tahl Dance Academy
182 High Street
Nutley, NJ 07110
(201) 667-3223

Sahda's Centre for
the Danse Orientale
(Lynda Mathé)
505 Allwood Road
Clifton, NJ 07012
(201) 778-8652

Tara's Belly Dance Studios
618 6th Avenue
Lyndhurst, NJ 07071
(201) 933-9331

New Mexico

Alia's School of
Middle Eastern Dance
1313 Mesa Verde
Farmington, NM 87401
(505) 325-7147

New York

Angelica Dance Studio
Ballet Academy
195 Willis Avenue
Mineola, NY 11501
(516) 717-8212

Arabesque Studio (Ayesha)
Box 270
Syosset, NY 11791
(516) 365-1869

Belly's Dance Studio
37-11 Union Street
Flushing, NY 11354
(212) 445-9392

Cia Cirel Studio 4
317 Sixth Avenue
New York, NY 10014
(212) 929-2326

Elektra's Home of
Middle Eastern Dance
163 Anchorage Drive
West Islip, NY 11795
(516) 587-2863

Ibrahim Farrah
Instructor of Near Eastern
Dance Arts
Choreographer/Director
The Near East Dance Group
Publisher of Arabesqué
One Sherman Square, Suite 22 F
New York, NY 10023
(212) 595-1677

International Dance Studio
Studio 819, Carnegie Hall
881 7th Avenue
New York, NY 10019
(212) 247-6056

Lee Fox Sheldon Dance Studio
66 North Lane
Angola, NY 14006
(716) 549-2616

Morocco
Mideastern Dance Academy
150 West 75th Street #9
New York, NY 10023
(212) 799-1272 or 580-2731

Navida
P. O. Box 247
Lenox Hill Station
New York, NY 10021
(212) 737-0209

Nyeelah's School of
Middle Eastern Dance
Judy Goldberg
348 North Columbus Avenue
Mt. Vernon, NY 10552
(914) 668-8772

Regine Middle Eastern
Oriental Dancing
894 South Long Branch Avenue
Freeport, NY 11520
(516) 623-4789

Scheherazade's School of
Mid-East Dance
20 Dunham Road
Hartsdale, NY 10530
(914) 693-2181

Stephania Studios
10 Martine Avenue
White Plains, NY 10601
(914) 949-1220

Valerie Leopold Dance Workshop
295 Culver Parkway
Rochester, NY 14609
(716) 288-4090 or 288-3394

Ohio

Dance Du Ventre
6117 Teagarden Circle
Dayton, OH 45449
(513) 435-0824

Ellen Deaton (Schehera)
2518 Salem Avenue (Rt. 49)
Dayton, OH 45406
(513) 277-9195

Habeeba's Dance of the Arts, Inc.
2650 North High Street
Columbus, OH 43202
(614) 267-2514 or 267-2515
Other Locations: Cincinnati,
Columbus East, Marion,
Circleville, Chillicothe,
Newark, Marysville

Sabiha's School of
Middle Eastern Dance, Inc.
80 Mill Street
Athens, OH 45701
(614) 592-4085

Oklahoma

Elona
4304 S. Louisville Avenue
Tulsa, OK 74135
(918) 749-7255

Oregon

Celaeno's
P. O. Box 22372
Milwaukie, OR 97222
(503) 654-1101

Pennsylvania

Joyce Freeman Studio of Dance
2709 South Queen Street
York, PA 17403
(717) 244-2420 or 741-2272

Marika's School of
Mid-Eastern Dance
2328 Grandview Boulevard
Reading, PA 19609
(215) 678-7122

Shia Vazon
6103 West Mill Road
Flourtown, PA 19031
(215) 836-5359

Texas

Bacchanal School of Belly Dance
Dir. George Garifallos
(Mahal, Instructor)
535 Westheiner
Houston, TX 77006
(713) 527-0944

Mahal Academy of Belly Dancing
Dir. George Garifallos
(Mahal, Instructor)
1371 South Voss
Houston, TX 77057
(713) 977-1628

Meara School of Dance
5621 Alpha Road
Dallas, TX 75240
(214) 661-3734

Virginia

Sheva's School of Belly Dancing
6603 Juniper Street
Richmond, VA 23230
(804) 266-6900

Washington

Charlotte Peppel
Directress of Academy of Dance
2821 Wetmore Avenue
Everett, WA 98201
(206) 252-7487

Diane Edrington
Tacoma Community College
5900 South 12th Street
Tacoma, WA 98465
(206) 756-5000

Kathleen's School of Dance
707 "J" St.
Seventh Street Theater
Hoquiam, WA 98550
(206) 532-7109

Saadia Latifa
Middle Eastern Dance
Instructions
20113 68th Avenue W.
Lynwood, WA 98036
(206) 776-1266

West Virginia

Jeanny's Oriental Exercises
and Dances
101 Cherry Drive
Shinnston, WV 26431
(304) 592-3931

Wisconsin

Balkula's
3907 North 84th Street
Milwaukee, WI 53222
(414) 461-8350

Pat Kellar Dance Studio
9207 West Center Street
Milwaukee, WI 53222
(404) 774-0620 or 786-6933

Tara (The Original)
Tara's School of Dance
1709 Monroe Street
Madison, WI 53711
(608) 255-4444

Canada

Dance Orientale School
Master Teacher &
Artistic Director, Diane Calenti
100 Richmond Street East
Suite 309
Toronto M5C1P1, Canada
(416) 368-8412

Freddy's Dancing Academy
Director—Prof. Eddy Manneh
165 Bloor Street East
Toronto, Ontario, Canada
(416) 925-2288

ORIENTAL DANCE COSTUMES AND ACCESSORIES FROM A TO Z

California

Jodette's Belly Dancing Academy
P. O. Box 9024
Sacramento, CA 95816
(916) 929-8429
or 447-0637
(A very complete offering of
items for the
Oriental dancer)

Persian Bazaar
107 Serramonte Center
Daly City, CA 94015
(415) 994-2010
(Everything for the dancer)

Sula's Belly Dance World
1235 Boulevard Way
Walnut Creek, CA 94595
(415) 937-7852

Yasmen Bovée
P. O. Box 99152
San Diego, CA 92109
(714) 286-2375
(Books, Records, Cymbals)

Florida

Juliana Dance Gallery
102 Giralda
Coral Gables, FL 33134
(305) 448-6420
(Art photographs, Custom-
designed tables, lamps, room
dividers, Natural form
jewelry)

The Spotlight
2754 North Federal Highway
Fort Lauderdale, FL 33306
(305) 564-7722
(Oriental dance items)

World Gifts
557 Dodecanese Boulevard
Tarpon Springs, FL 33589
(813) 938-2211

Illinois

Beverly Rare Records
Novelty and Costume Shop
11612 S. Western Avenue
Chicago, IL 60643
(312) 779-0066

Melanie Sanford
856 N. Spring Street
Elgin, IL 60120
(312) 888-1103
(Costumes, Zills, Records)

Indiana

Dorvana's Mideast-Wear House
and Navel Academy
1503 E. Riverside Drive
Indianapolis, IN 46202
(317) 846-1921

Massachusetts

Acme T. V. Supply Co.
615 Mt. Auburn Street
Watertown, MA 02172
(617) 926-0450
(Headquarters for Oriental dance
and Near Eastern tapes and
records, Finger Cymbals, etc.)

Missouri

Opal's Belly Dance World
P. O. Box 20199
St. Louis, MO 63123
(314) 843-8282 or 843-1931
(Records)

New Jersey

Penny Lo Bello
Mid-East School of Dance
81 Cortlandt Place
Tenafly, NJ 07670
(201) 569-2225
(Costumes)

New York

Zahra Kader
429 West 43rd Street
New York, NY 10019
(212) 246-2736
(Custom Costumes)

Cheenavida Designs
P. O. Box 247
Lenox Hill Station
New York, NY 10021
(212) 737-0209
(Oriental dance skirts,
Accessories, Custom-designed
costumes, Egyptian belledi shifts)

The Dance Mart
Box 48, Homecrest Station
Brooklyn, NY 11229
(212) 627-0477
(Mail order dance books)

Guriak Records
276 Fifth Avenue
New York City, NY 10001
(212) 683-6111
(Complete assortment of
Middle Eastern and Armenian
recordings, tapes, records,
books, zills, etc.)

Rashid Sales Co.
191 Atlantic Avenue
Brooklyn, NY 11201
(212) UL 2-3295/8
(Records, Vast selection of
Arabic books)

Sahadi Importing Co., Inc.
187 Atlantic Avenue
Brooklyn, NY 11201
(212) 624-4550
(Belly dance costumes and
accessories)

North Carolina

Reznicks Inc.
Thruway Shopping Center
Winston-Salem, NC 27103
(919) 723-9735
(Records, 8-Track tapes)

Ohio

Ellis Bakery
577 Grant Street
Akron, OH 44311
(216) 376-5022
(Zills, durbakkeh drums;
Turkish pipes, Syrian cook books)

Ridge Records
Parmatown Shopping Center
7421 Ridgewood Drive
Parma, OH 44129
(216) 885-0160
(Records)

Oregon

Celaeno's
P. O. Box 22372
Milwaukie, OR 97222
(503) 654-1101
(Custom costumes)

Pennsylvania

Jamil Metal Products Co.
2328 Grandview Boulevard
Reading, PA 19609
(215) 678-7122
(Zills)

Washington

Continental Pastry
4549 University Way N.E.
Seattle, WA 98105
(206) 632-4700
(Mid-Eastern items, Records,
Pastries, Cymbals)

Wisconsin

Grecian Imports
4819 West North Avenue
Milwaukee, WI 53208
(414) 871-3780
(Authentic reproductions of
Greek art crafts, Jewelry)

Topping and Co.—
The International House
736 North 2nd Street
Milwaukee, WI 53203
(414) 272-2995
(Imported foods, Navel service,
Records)

PUBLICATIONS

Arabesque
A Journal of Middle Eastern
Dance and Culture
Ibrahim Farrah Inc.
One Sherman Square
Suite 22F
New York, NY 10023

Habibi Publications
P. O. Box 4081
Mt. View, CA 94040

The Belly Dancer Magazine
Yasmeen Samra
Editor/Publisher
P. O. Box 321
Los Altos, CA 94022

ORIENTAL DANCE RECORDS

A

A Night in the Middle East—Vol. 1—Ray Mirijanian and his Middle Eastern Ensemble—Magnasound Recording Studio

A Night in the Middle East—Vol. 3—Ray Mirijanian and his Middle Eastern Ensemble—Mirta Records

Alla Turca—The Turkish Way with Ozel—Tarik Bulut—Elay Records

Arabesque—Vol. 1—Traditional & Folk Dances of the Near East—Orient Records

Arabesque—Vol. 2—Authentic Oriental Dance Tempos—Orient Records

Arabian Delight—Abdu-El-Hanid and his Orchestra—Monitor

Arabic Songs of Lebanon and Egypt—George Sewaya Trio and Female Chorus—Folkways

Artistic Moods for Dance—Fred Elias & John Tatassopoulas—Intrasonic

B

Babylon Mood—Munir Bechir and his Quartet—A Chahine & Fils, Beirut

Bedouin Belly Dance—Youssef Kassab—Peters International

Bedouin Romance—Samira Tawfiq & Fahd Ballon—Voix Du Liban

Belly Dance—Spectacular Rhythms from Middle East—Peters International

Belly Dance for Arabian Nights—Abbud Abdel Aal and his Golden Strings—Peters International

Belly Dance Music—The "Flames of Araby Orchestra"—Vocals by George Abdo—Monitor

Belly Dance with Omar Karshid and his Magic Guitar—Parlophone

Belly Dancing at the Feenjon—The Feenjon Group—Monitor

Belly Dancing for Everyone—Chris Kalogerson—Monitor

Belly Dancing with George Abdo—Monitor

C

Cafe Feenjon Featuring the Feenjon Group—Menachem Dworman—Fran Records

Cafe Telaviv Featuring Jimmy Linardos and his Near-East Group—Fran Records

Caravan–Melodies of the Middle East—Abood Abdel Aal—Orient Record Company

D

Dabkie—Exotic Dances of the Middle East—The Derbecke Ensemble—American-London Series

Dance Into Your Sultan's Heart—Ozel—Elay Records

Dance of the Harem—Authentic Arab Music—A Chahine & Fils—Emi Parlophone

Dances of Port Said—Music of the Middle East—Mahammed El Bakkar and his Oriental Ensemble—Vol. 5—Audio Fidelity

Dark Eyes and Oriental Moods—Peters International

E

El Layalli El Hilwa—Orient Recording Company

Exciting Moods from Mid East—Harry Minasian—Scepter

Exotic Belly Dancers—Tat'Oul Al'Toun Middle East Ensemble—Guirak Records

H

How to Belly Dance for Your Sultan—Ozel—Elay Records

How to Make Your Husband a Sultan—Belly Dance With Ozel Turkbas—Elay Records

I

Istanbul—Authentic Music of the Near East—Authentic Orchestras and Soloists of the Near East—Standard Phono Corp.

J

Jimmy Leonardos and his Orchestra—Mid East Music with Three Routines

Jimmy Linardos and his Near-East Group Invite You to Belly Dance—Vol. 1—An Isaac Hager Production—Fran Records

K

Karizma Teaches Belly Dancing—An Instructional Record

Kef Time Detroit—Group #31—Buddy Sarkissian, Richard A. Hagopian—Saha Records

Kef Time Fresno

Kef Time Hartford

Kef Time Las Vegas

L

Lebanon—Baalbek Folk Festival featuring Fairouz—Monitor

Little Egypt Presents How to Belly Dance for Your Husband—Sonny Lester Orch.—Roulette Records

M

Mater Plays His Magic Bouzouki—Only for a King—Voice of Stars

Middle East Hit Parade—Romel Lahoud—Monitor

Middle Eastern Caravan—Eddie Kochak & Souren Baranian & Mid Eastern Ensemble—Guirak Records

Middle Eastern Soul—Bob Tashjian, Souren Baronian with the Mid-Eastern Ensemble—Carlee Records

Music for Belly Dancing—Anestos Atheunasiou and his Ensemble—Monitor

Music for an Oriental Dance—*Vol. 1*—Rafik Hobeika—Voice of Lebanon

Music for an Oriental Dance—*Vol. 2*—*Rafik* Hobeika—Voice of Lebanon

Music of the Near East and Middle East—*The Oud*—Aram Gulezian and his Orchestra—Lyricord

N

Nadira Belly Dances for Youssef Kassab—Youssef Kassab—Peters International

O

Ode To An Oud—John Berberian—Mainstream (2-record set)

O Ilios Tis Anatolis—*Turkish Belly Dance*—Peters International

Oriental Nights—Mohamed Madi Orchestra—Monitor

P

Picture Yourself Belly Dancing—The Topkapi Instrumental Ensemble—Monitor

Port Said—*Music of the Middle East*—Mohammed El-Bakkar and his Oriental Ensemble—Audio Fidelity

Q

Queen of Dancers—Iklas Osman—Cinera-Phone

S

Soraya My Love—*Songs from the Middle East*—Soraya Melik—Monitor

Strictly Belly Dancing—*Vols. 1 through 6*—Eddie "The Sheik" Kochak—West End Music

T

Takseem "Improvisation"—Authentic Instrumental Music by the most Famous Arab Artists—Ash-Shark Records

Ten Dynamic Nights from Thousand and One Nights—Voice of Stars Records

The Art of Belly Dancing—George Abdo and his "Flames of Araby" Orchestra—Monitor

The Joy of Belly Dancing—George Abdo and his "Flames of Araby" Orchestra—Monitor

Turkish Delight—Mike Sarkissian and his Bagdad Ensemble—Audio Fidelity

Turkish Delight—New Sounds from the Near East—The Dolgru Yol Turkish Ensemble—Monitor

Dance teachers may contact Monitor Recordings Inc. directly at 156 Fifth Avenue, New York, 10010

SLOW TUNES FOR YOUR EXERCISES

Record	Side	Tune
Alla Turca	2	Salla, Salla
	2	Improvisations (floor work)
A Night in the Middle East	1	Hala Laya
	2	Aman Koyzoym, Aman Koyzoym
	2	Al Asfooreyeh
	2	Erev Shelshoshanim
Babylon Mood	1	Meshwar Ma'Al Oud—A Promenade with the Aoud (good for mind and body preparedness)
Ode To An Oud—Record #1	1	Bir Demet Yasemen
	1	Savgulum
	2	Yarus
	2	Rast Taksim (floor work)
Ode To An Oud—Record #2	1	Basha Bella
	2	Taksim (floor work)
Reflections of the Near East	B	Danse Arabe

Strictly Belly Dancing		
Ya Habibi #2, Vol. 1	A	Cleopatra
	A	Chifte Telle (floor work)
	B	Chutak Melody (fast ending)
	B	Shifte Armany
	B	Oud Fantasy (floor work)
Strictly Belly Dancing,	1	The Sensual Chifti
Vol. 2.	2	Ya-Bul-Ayoun-Il-Sood
	2	Sel-Im-Alay
	2	Ya-Mali-Sham
The Art of Belly Dancing	1	Raks Al-Sultan
	2	Raks Pharonic
	2	Gameel Gamal
The Joy of Belly Dancing	1	Raks Abdo
	1	Raks El Gezlan
	1	Miserlou
	2	Raks Leyla
	2	A Nada
Turkish Delight	1	Chifte Telli

FAST TUNES FOR YOUR EXERCISES

Record	*Side*	*Tune*
Alla Turca	2	Bride From Bursa
	2	Keep Dancing, Keep Turning
	2	The Camel Driver
A Night in the Middle East	1	Doktor
	1	Siselar
	2	Arabaya Tas Koydum (Karslimar)
	2	Ah Ya Zein
Ode to an Oud—	1	Aziza
Record #1	2	Sevasda
Ode to an Oud—	1	Siseler
Record #2	2	Arabaya (starts slow)
	2	Whyek
Reflections of the Near East	A	Sobhano
	A	Yahdein
	A	El Mataam
	A	Mahma Kount
	B	Al Bourj

Strictly Belly Dancing		
Ya Habibi #2, Vol. 1	A	Ma Elee
	A	Ah Yah Zein
	B	Kadife (Karslimar)
	B	Wedding Party
Strictly Belly Dancing,	1	Leila
Vol. 2	2	Hamil Ya Ghanam
The Art of Belly Dancing	1	Raks Musri (fast, slow, fast)
	1	Meenie Yaba
	1	Raks Araby
	1	Raks Al-Dounya
The Joy of Belly Dancing	1	Noora Ya Noora
	2	Raks Averof (fast, then slow)
Turkish Delight	1	Darling One
	1	I Gave a Handkerchief to the Bride (Karslimar)
	1	Nino Nino
	1	Do You Want Ali, My Daughter

MIDDLE EASTERN AND GREEK FOOD SHOPS

Alabama

Lignos Grocery
160 Government Street
Mobile, AL
(205) 432-9870

Arizona

Little Greek Shop
1135 East Glendale Avenue
Phoenix, AZ 85020
(602) 625-7669

California

Bezjian's Grocery
4725 Santa Monica Blvd.
Hollywood, CA 90029
(213) 663-1503

C & K Importing Co.
2771 West Pico Blvd.
Los Angeles, CA 90006
(213) 737-2970

International Delicatessen
265 East 18th Street
Oakland, CA 94606
(415) 451-8337

S & J Importing Co.
1770 Pacific Avenue
Long Beach, CA 90813
(213) 599-1341

Connecticut

Dimyanis Market
116 Elm Street
Danbury, CT 06810
(203) 748-3747

Steve's Market
157 Washington Street
South Norwalk, CT 06854
(203) 853-4020

Delaware

Calavrita Importing Co., Inc.
12 East Fourth Street
Wilmington, DE 19801
(302) 654-1624

District of Columbia

Acropolis Food Market
1206 Underwood Street, N.W.
Washington, D. C. 20012
(202) 829-1414 or (202) 829-1415

Hellas Greek Import
1245 20th Street, N.W.
Washington, D.C. 20036
(202) 785-0861

Skenderis
1612 20th Street, N.W.
Washington, D. C. 20009
(202) 265-9664-7

Florida

Alex Bakery Corp.
878 S. W. 8th Street
Miami, Florida 33130
(305) 858-4218

Greek American Grocery Co.
2690 S. W. 22nd Street
Miami, FL 33145

Mercury's Imp. Food Market
501 North Pinellas Avenue
Tarpon Springs, FL 33589
(813) 937-3704

Illinois

Columbus Food Mart & Bakery
1651 Rand Road
Des Plaines, IL 60016
(312) 297-6660

International Foods, Inc.
4724 North Kedzie Avenue
Chicago, IL 60625
(312) 478-8643

International Foods, N.W., Inc.
4404 West Fullerton
Chicago, IL 60639
(321) 486-6277

International Foods, West, Inc.
3417 West Diversey Avenue
Chicago, IL 60647
(312) 384-0959

Sparta Grocery
6050 West Diversey Avenue
Chicago, IL 60639
(312) 637-8073

Kentucky

A. Thomas & Sons, Meat Co.
Haymarket Square
309 East Jefferson Street
Louisville, KY 40202
(502) 587-6947

Louisiana

Central Grocery Co.
923 Decatur Street
New Orleans, LA 70116
(504) 523-1620

Maryland

Skenderis
5558 Randolph Road
Rockville, MD 20852
(301) 770-5558

Thomas Market
2650 University Blvd. West
Wheaton, MD 20902
(301) 942-0839

Massachusetts

Syrian Grocery Importing Co.
270 Shawmut Avenue
Boston, MA 02118
(617) 338-9657

Michigan

Mediterranean Grocery
11431 West Jefferson Avenue
River Rouge, MI 48218
(313) 842-3270

New Jersey

Central Food Store
63 Main Street
Hackensack, NJ 07601
(201) 342-2113

Parthenon Gift Shop & Foods #1
344 Clifton Avenue
Clifton, NJ 07011
(201) 365-1810

Parthenon Gift & Food Shop #2
357 Fairview Avenue
Fairview, NJ 07021
(201) 945-0871
(201) 945-9641

New York

Baruir's Oriental-American
Grocery
40-07 Queens Blvd.
Sunnyside, NY 11104
(212) 784-0842

Damascus Bakery Inc.
195 Atlantic Avenue
Brooklyn, NY 11201
(212) 855-1456

George Malko Importing Co.
182 Atlantic Avenue
Brooklyn, NY 11201
(212) 624-2049
(212) 624-2267

Grecian Products Inc.
7708 3rd Avenue
Brooklyn, NY 11209
(212) 836-8151

Karnig Tashjian
380 Third Avenue
New York, NY 10016
(212) 683-8458

Kassos Brothers
570 Ninth Avenue
New York, NY 10036
(212) 736-7473

Melkon Candy Co. Inc.
3074 31st Street
Astoria, NY 11102
(212) 278-9286

Sahadi Importing Co.
187 Atlantic Avenue
Brooklyn, NY 11201
(212) 624-4550

Thanos Imported Groceries
424 Pearl Street
Syracuse, NY 13203
(315) 422-4085

Ohio

Athens Pastry Shop, Inc.
2545 Lorain Avenue
Cleveland, OH 44113
(216) 861-8149

Ellis Bakery
577 Grant Street
Akron, OH 44311
(216) 376-5012

Olympic Imports
5435 Pearl Road
Parma, OH 44129
(216) 886-1668

Utah

Broadway Shopping Center
242 East 3rd South
Salt Lake City, UT 84111
(801) 363-3155
(801) 363-3939

Washington

Continental Pastry
4549 University Way, N.E.
Seattle, WA 98105
(206) 632-4700

West Virginia

R A Medovic
A. G. Food Center
2201 Market Street
Wheeling, WV 26003
(304) 232-1118

Wisconsin

Grecian Imports
4819 West North Avenue
Milwaukee, WI 53208
(414) 871-3480

Topping & Co.—
The International House
736 North Second Street
Milwaukee, WI 53203
(414) 272-2995

INDEX